Full
Strength

Full Strength

A Training Handbook for a Strong Back
and a Healthy Body

Werner Kieser

Kieser Training
Zurich
Switzerland

MARTIN DUNITZ

© Copyright 2000 by Werner Kieser
© Copyright of original German publication 2000 by Wilhelm Heyne Verlag GmbH & Co. KG, Munich

Kieser Training® is a registered trademark

Illustrations by Holger Vanselow, Hamburg
Photographs by Silvia Volpi, Zurich

This translation © Martin Dunitz 2002

Translated by Sue Coles

First published in the United Kingdom by
Martin Dunitz Ltd, The Livery House, 7–9 Pratt Street, London NW1 0AE

Tel: +44 (0)20 7482 2202
Fax: +44 (0)20 7482 7088
E-mail: info.dunitz@tandf.co.uk
Website: www.dunitz.co.uk

A CIP catalogue record for this book is available from the British Library

ISBN 1-84184-094-7

Distributed in the USA by
Fulfilment Center
Taylor & Francis
7625 Empire Drive
Florence, KY 41042, USA
Toll Free Tel: 1-800-634-7064
Email: cserve@routledge_ny.com

Distributed in Canada by
Taylor & Francis
74 Rolark Drive
Scarborough
Ontario M1R G2, Canada
Toll Free Tel: 1-877-226-2237
Email: tal_fran@istar.ca

Distributed in the rest of the world by
ITPS Limited
Cheriton House
North Way, Andover
Hampshire SP10 5BE, UK
Tel: +44- (0)1264 332424
Email: reception@itps.co.uk

Composition by Scribe Design, Gillingham, Kent, UK
Printed and bound in Spain by Estudios Graficos ZURE

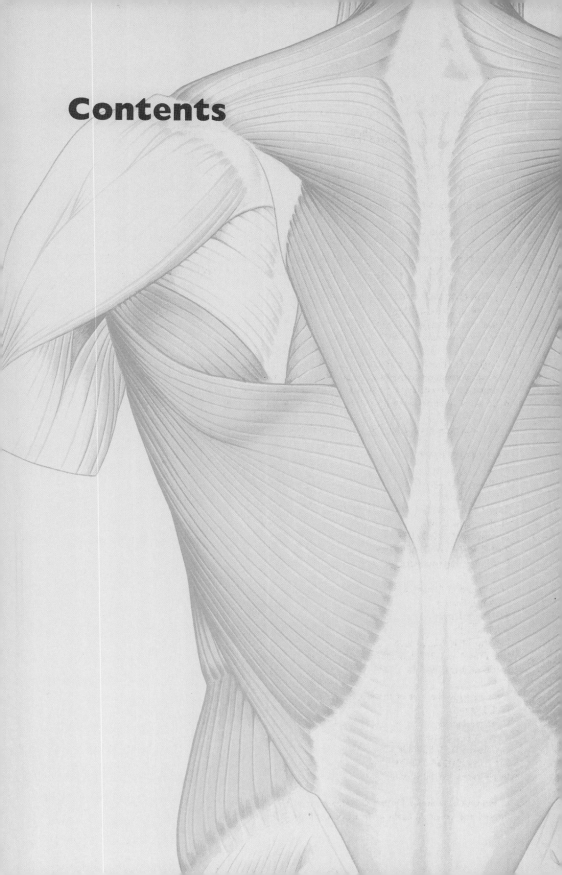

Contents

Preface

We live in an ageing, backward-looking society with a yearning for youth. Many take up a sport not because of a desire to achieve something tangible but simply because they want to be part of the "in" crowd. Today we can buy into any given "lifestyle". A lifestyle manifests itself in our clothes, hairstyle, car, our furniture and membership of exclusive and sometimes not so exclusive clubs. However, what we buy is often nothing more than a substitute for a more fundamental change in the way we live. It is wrong to complain that society has become more "narcissistic" or "egotistic". In fact the opposite is true: such pseudo-effort (it is not effort in the true sense of the word) is designed to "create a personal image". It is an example of opportunistic behaviour. It is self-denial in its literal sense, a form of indulgence perpetuated by the fear that we might suddenly be "out". We are unable to drop this pretence and so lose our ability to look at facts objectively.

For example getting older is an undeniable fact of life. Even if we wear a youthful ponytail or drive a sports car we still get older. The fact that we can do something to prevent one of the main problems associated with old age — weak muscles — is still largely unknown. Perhaps this is because it is not something we can merely buy. It requires us to do something.

Another unpopular fact is that there is relatively little we can do to change our body. The flood of advertising makes us believe that we can all be thin, beautiful, desirable and successful. All that is required is a firm belief and then to buy the relevant product. However, the way we look and what we achieve is largely determined by our genetic makeup. We cannot change our body size or proportions: the relationship between leg length and body. Similarly our potential to increase strength through training or exercises to improve dexterity is predetermined. The location and nature of fat accumulation, our sensory and intellectual abilities, such as musical ability, mathematical talent, are also predetermined: all facts that we would prefer to forget in favour of a more alluring way of looking at things.

We are at the mercy of a sales industry that devotes itself to that tenet of modern marketing. "If you want it, we can supply it!" It may hide behind a hackneyed expression such as "holistic" but what it really means is that a buyer can be found for almost every conceivable idiocy.

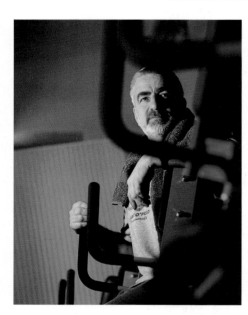

In a market based on aspirations and promises it is not easy to gain an audience for a concept based on reality. Having been disappointed so many times consumers have become sceptical.

When I first started to take a close look at strength training the term did not even exist. Even students training to be sports teachers regarded strength as merely something of interest to weightlifters. However, today strength training is an accepted part of their syllabus—a welcome development but merely a beginning. Many are still unaware that the benefits to be derived from preventive and medical strength training are almost limitless.

Almost every day I receive letters from people who thank their lucky stars that they discovered strength training by pure chance. The aim of this book is to give chance a helping hand.

Werner Kieser

Why we need strength

You need strength as soon as you wake up. Without it you would be unable even to get out of bed. Imagine waking up one day to find that you had lost 50% of your weight overnight without any loss of strength. It would feel as if you were gliding out of bed.

Muscles (and only muscles) are what allow you to move. Muscles support you and it is their strength that determines whether you enjoy life or find it a physical chore. Muscles also determine whether you suffer from back pain. They determine whether you have that nagging feeling that you ought to be doing "something" about your figure or whether you (and others) are satisfied with yourself as you now are.

Without the strength of your muscles you cannot move

What is strength training?

Because athletes were the first to take up strength training many people still regard it as a sporting discipline, but it is not. Strength training is a rational way of improving your physical performance. Similarly it is not an adjunct to a sport but its essence. Strength training embraces in a single discipline the benefits of a sport that we consider "healthy". Irrespective of what sport you choose, what improves your physical appearance is your increase in strength.

How do we increase muscle strength? Many cling to the idea that all that is needed is some form of movement. That is why there is so much talk about the "lack of movement" from which we allegedly suffer. However, in reality we lack not movement but resistance. Most movements are done against a random resistance, primarily the Earth's gravitational pull. These movements may have a training effect but it is not inevitable that they will.

What we lack is not movement but resistance

This is why actual movement is secondary in strength training. What counts is resistance. Machine-based training allows us to dispense the right level of

Strength training
changes our physical
appearance

resistance, to control the path of that resistance, to distinguish between real and pseudo-progress and to record such progress. Strength training is not particularly fun. Similarly it is not that good for developing social contacts. If that is the case why do so many do it? Because it works! No other method produces such fundamental and externally visible changes to our appearance.

Benefits of strength training

Training prevents
physical degeneration

Health-oriented strength training improves the basic physical condition. If you are still young strong muscles act as a natural "corset", that supports and carries you throughout your life. If you are older it retards physical degeneration and accelerates regeneration.

Reduces effect of gravity

Training increases strength and so improves the strength to weight ratio. Remember that muscle strength is all that keeps you upright, gets you upstairs and supports you. Without muscle strength you would be unable to move, at least not without external help. Why do we feel so good in the bath? It is because the displacement of water gives us a feeling of almost total weightlessness. With strength training you can experience this feeling all the time, making it easier to support your body weight.

Improves appearance

The condition and shape of your muscles are what determine your external appearance, including the way you move. Flabby untrained muscles make you look flabby. Everything tends to sag. Exercise improves muscle tone and with it your figure.

Improves flexibility

Machine-based strength training puts a load on a muscle in both its extended and contracted state. It is, therefore, more effective at increasing mobility than traditional exercises. If we contract one muscle fully this in turn means that we extend its antagonist fully (for example, biceps/triceps).

Eliminates back pain

Weak back muscles are the cause of 80% of back problems. A strong back knows no pain. Recent research has shown that targeted strength training is the only effective way to prevent and treat back problems. Passive measures (fango treatments, medicinal baths, etc.) aggravate symptoms in the long term.

Strong back muscles prevent pain

Prevents osteoporosis

It is not just muscles and tendons that respond to resistance. Bones also become stronger.

Speeds up recovery

Strength training stimulates anabolic processes and so reduces recovery time considerably, such as after surgery. Each muscle is more or less isolated and then exercised separately. This means that training can continue even if individual limbs are immobilized, for example, in plaster.

Improves protection against injury

Training increases the density and specific weight of a muscle and so improves defences in the event of an external impact (armour function).

Helps you lose weight more efficiently

If you use more calories than you consume the body has to draw on its own resources and you lose both fat and muscle. This is why those on starvation diets often look worse than they did before. However, if strength training is done at the same time the muscle is retained and fat is shed more quickly. Muscles are good fat burners.

Increases self-confidence

The changes brought about by strength training are greater than you would expect. It makes you more relaxed. It develops a feeling of inner self-confidence, which in turn improves your inter-personal skills.

Improves posture

Strength training corrects imbalances

Poor posture is the result of an imbalance in inter-muscular tension. The stresses and strains of daily life, physical labour and even the sports we play all have a one-sided effect. Strength training corrects these imbalances.

Retains strength in old age

We cannot stop the passage of time but we can prevent increasing weakness. A prime cause of the infirmities of old age is loss of muscle and bone tissue and with it strength. We lose control over our body. This makes us anxious. The risk of fractures is also higher. Strength training helps increase and maintain strength and so we retain control over our body.

How does strength training work?

We have all witnessed the process at work on our own body. If we damage our skin the process of healing continues even after the injury has healed. Tissue continues to form in the area of damaged skin. The result is a scar with the skin remaining somewhat thicker than before the injury. A similar process takes place after a fracture or a serious loss of blood. Scientists refer to this as an "excess reaction". Apparently nature builds up tissue in order to protect against future damage.

Nature wards off possible damage by increasing tissue growth

"Supercompensation" is the term used to describe the response of living organisms to an increased load; that is, they increase their own reserves.

Strength training exploits this principle. If you subject a muscle to an unusually high load it initially

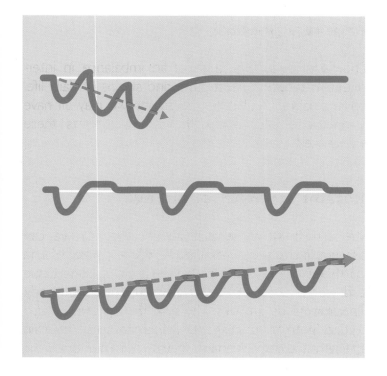

Top: if interval is too short there is a rapid decrease in strength.

Middle: if interval is too long we lose the training gain before we train next time.

Bottom: if the interval is correct strength increases incrementally.

Overtraining
weakens muscles

loses, but then increases, its strength. However, the reaction is not immediate. If the recovery time is too short, for instance, if we train too often, we not only weaken our muscles but we weaken ourselves as well. "Overtraining" is particularly damaging to our immune system.

Strength training and competitive sport

Even 30 years ago strength training was either unknown or at least most trainers were suspicious of it. It was thought that "too much" strength would reduce the flexibility and speed of athletes. However, it soon became clear to even the most adamant critics of strength training that all other things being equal the honours would go to the strongest—and this applied whatever the sport. But what are these "other things"?

Inherited attributes

If you are only 5 feet tall you could play basketball every day for 30 years and still not be a top player. Similarly, despite muscles like Arnold Schwarzenegger you will never be a good weightlifter if you have long legs and arms. If your legs are relatively short compared with your trunk, a career as say a high jumper is out of the question. If the length of your muscle belly (central fleshy part of muscle between tendon transitions) is relatively short compared with tendon length, your capacity to increase muscle size is so limited that even with all the training and chemicals in the world you will never be a bodybuilding champion.

Competitive athletes are a genetic elite with certain innate attributes. Although this is of interest to trainers and scientists, it has no bearing on health. Perhaps 1 in 10,000 men has the genetic potential to develop the muscles required for a "Mr Universe". Apart from a physical predisposition, many sports also require neuro-physiological skills such as rapid reactions.

The ratio between muscle length and tendon length determines the potential for muscle growth

Environment

Childhood experiences, education, social environment and our social system mould our moral attitudes and in turn our character. Determination and tenacity (as character traits) can undoubtedly improve sporting achievement. However, they are only effective if combined with the required predisposition.

Success in sport requires a certain predisposition

Coordination

However good your predisposition you can only exploit it if you practise. Herein lies mankind's greatest reserve. The majority of movements you do, whether as a shot-putter, boxer or pianist, require coordination. Coordination refers to the way our nervous system controls muscle movements. We tend to take movements like standing up, walking or sitting down for granted. However, if you look more closely you will find that they are a highly complicated set of individual movements synchronized with extreme precision by our nervous system and involving a chain of muscles each working to a greater or lesser extent. We learn these patterns of movement and then by frequent repetition eliminate any unnecessary movement. We store these "established patterns" in the brain from where they can be accessed as kinetic memory patterns. They are called engrams, specific "interconnections". Once in our memory we find these movements easy and can do them without thinking. It may take some effort to learn the movement in the first place but from then on it is automatic.

Coordination is the control of muscles by the nervous system

Movement patterns are task-specific and are not transferable to other similar tasks. For example the best form of "practice" for a footballer is football. If his training regime includes other activities that require coordination, for example, steeplechasing, cycling or swimming they will not help his abilities on the pitch.

Does strength change your style?

Prejudice dies hard. There are still coaches who fear that strength training will harm athletes. However, it has been found that their concerns are largely unjustified. Strength training improves flexibility and speed. Nevertheless a certain degree of caution is not totally inappropriate because changes in strength also change the strength statics of the musculoskeletal system, which may—at least in the short term—have a negative effect on athletic performance. Why?

Strength training improves mobility and speed

The way we move—our style—is the result and expression of the ratio of strength between one muscle and another. Very often we tend to favour our stronger muscles over our weaker muscles. We adapt to our own strengths and weaknesses and create our own style. If these strength ratios are changed, either up or down, certain movement patterns become redundant or are no longer appropriate. It may take several months to learn new patterns and during the transitional phase coordination is sub-optimal.

We tend to use stronger muscles and spare weaker ones

Imagine if your income doubled almost overnight. Your lifestyle would change only gradually. However, after some time you would settle into the "high life". A similar thing happens with strength. If you double your strength you continue to move for some time as though you were still weaker, that is, you do not make full use of your new resources. However, once your coordination has adapted to the new level of strength the problem disappears.

Do not confuse strength with co-ordination

Mention must be made here of a popular method of sports training, which despite its popularity is totally misguided. I am referring to the method of imitating movements in a particular sport but doing them under more difficult conditions. In an endeavour to offer practical training some coaches recommend that javelin throwers use a heavier javelin in practice in the hope that their protégés will become stronger and so throw the normal lighter javelin much further. Similarly some high-jumpers wear a vest filled with a lead weight. Sprinters have to overcome the resistance of a rubber strap before they can leave the starting block. However, as already indicated, movements are controlled by extremely complex processes that depend upon a constant set of external conditions. If you practise such movements under more difficult conditions you gradually develop new memory patterns. They will be slightly different from the "old" correct ones, such as those required in competition. The change, although slight, brings with it the risk of a "derailment": it can disrupt the movement patterns required in competition. In addition the strength increases achieved in this way are minimal because the load is spread over too many muscles and the tension in each muscle remains below the stimulus threshold.

Imitating movement patterns but with an additional load diminishes coordination and increases strength only slightly

Do competitive athletes need a special kind of strength training?

The use to which strength is put is of no relevance to a muscle. A muscle is in a delicate state of balance between strength build-up and strength loss and it either grows or does not grow. Strength build-up is not sport-specific even though many trainers think it is. There is only one type of strength not several. For both athletes and non-athletes the basic rule for strength training is short and intensive but not too often.

However, to train coordination the opposite is true: as often as possible but never to exhaustion, as otherwise you learn incorrect memory patterns.

Strength training is not sport-specific

Bodybuilding

A strong body is fashionable. The popularity of modern bodybuilding can be traced back to Hollywood and the film industry. When the first films were made about the Romans in the 1940s it soon became clear that there were few actors with the right physique.

In typical American fashion they were not prepared to make do with the "natural talent" that happened to be around. Rather they set about literally creating the required physique and so precipitated the global spread of bodybuilding. Bodybuilders set up national and international associations with their own aims and competition rules. The aim of bodybuilding is to develop each muscle to its full potential in order to maximize muscle contours. Competitors "pose" to demonstrate their level of muscle development and the winner is whosoever (from a visual perspective) displays not only the greatest but also the most balanced development. Judging is done by a panel of experts, similar to the method used in gymnastics and figure skating.

Bodybuilders seek to maximize muscle development

Bodybuilders use strength training to prepare for competition. They are concerned solely with external appearance, that is, visible muscle mass. They are not interested in considerations such as muscle function and health. Although bodybuilding concentrates solely on external appearance, it is one of the few sporting disciplines that is not harmful to health. The fact that bodybuilding is often combined with drug abuse is a

With bodybuilding the visible muscle mass is all that matters

quite different matter: it is a problem affecting all top sportsmen and women irrespective of their sport.

Strength training for heart and circulation

The exercise required to strengthen the heart muscle differs from that required for skeletal muscles. The necessary tension is achieved by an increase in output. The heart has to pump more blood per second and responds by increasing its volume, similar to the process with skeletal muscles. As a result the efficiency of respiratory muscles is also improved, the tidal volume is increased. The number of blood vessels increases and with it the volume of circulating blood. The heart is the most important muscle of all. If it fails death is instantaneous.

The heart is the most important muscle in the body

In response to the widespread incidence of circulatory ailments, specialists in preventive medicine have consistently drawn attention over the last 20 years to the need for and benefits of stamina training. The importance of strength training for both prevention and therapy—particularly for older men and women (osteoporosis) — is a relatively recent discovery and has yet to reach all doctors working in primary care. Stamina training is nothing more than strength training for the heart. Like any other muscle the response of the heart muscle to an increase in tension is to increase its strength. The heart achieves this level of tension if it has to pump round more blood. The pulse rate serves as a measurement. The current recommendation for the pulse rate is 170 beats per minute less half your age; this is the intensity you should maintain for 15–20 minutes two or three times a week. How you increase your pulse rate is not important. It can be done by cycling, running, swimming,

Cardiovascular training is strength training for the heart

skipping or even strength training. An excellent and safe way to exercise the heart is to walk uphill.

The most practical thing to do is to train strength and stamina simultaneously

Undoubtedly the most efficient and also the least harmful way is to combine stamina and strength training. The method is extremely simple—just keep the interval between each exercise to less than 15 seconds wherever possible.

Slim and supple

There is still a widespread belief that you can target where you lose weight: women generally want to lose it from their hips and thighs and men from their stomachs. This belief guarantees the continued existence of institutions that make promises to this effect. It is also why many "stomach" machines lie unused in cellars or attics. You cannot work off fat, melt it down, rub it away or even massage it off. Similarly abdominal exercises have no effect on abdominal fat. Where you accumulate fat is determined by your genetic makeup and cannot be controlled (except by the scalpel).

You cannot target where you lose weight

Fat is a reserve. You can only get rid of it by using it.

Fat does several jobs

Nature is ignorant of fashion. Layers of fat can be very useful in certain circumstances, for instance, if food supplies are uncertain or irregular. Then it makes sense to stock up and to store what is not needed immediately as fat layers.

Fatty tissue also provides protection against temperature changes. For example, long-distance swimmers develop a fat layer beneath the skin to protect them against hypothermia.

Your genes determine where you store fat. If you have blond hair and blue or green eyes you accumulate fat first in "niches" (such as the hollow behind the knee, the area between triceps and elbow, double chin, etc). After that fat reserves are deposited evenly over the surface of the body. In terms of geometry the body is like a sphere, that is, the shape with the smallest surface area to content ratio. This shape minimizes heat loss from the body, and in the regions where your ancestors came from—from the icy north—this was essential for survival.

Nature works in reverse for those with black hair, brown eyes and heavily pigmented skin. Such people concentrate fat deposits in a few prominent places (gluteal muscle, chest, and abdomen). This increases the surface area to content ratio, which allows heat to be emitted more quickly—very practical in hot countries. In other words the same material—body fat—can play contrasting roles. This genetic basis to fat accumulations also explains why you cannot control where you lose weight; you cannot lose it just where you want to.

Fat protects against cold and heat

Starvation diets are dangerous

If we take in more calories than we expend we put on weight. If we expend more calories than we take in we lose weight. It is as simple as that. In this context the quality of food is of secondary importance.

It makes little sense just to reduce food intake. Seventy percent of weight lost in this way is lost from muscles—the "load-bearing" substance. It has little effect on the substance "carried", that is, the fat. In other words it is a foolish thing to do and can be likened to burning the roof timbers to heat the house.

Similarly the other way of increasing calorie consumption, by doing more sport or general physical activity, makes little sense either. If you flood the

Starve yourself and you lose muscle not fat

bathroom it is not enough to mop up the water from the floor. You need to turn off the tap as well.

Exchange fat for muscle

If you are reducing your calorie intake you should also do strength training. This will prevent loss of strength and muscle. The aim here is not to increase calorie consumption—strength training only increases it slightly—but to force the body to change its priorities, that is, to lose fat and not muscle.

Strength training exerts a strong stimulus on anabolic processes, the physical processes responsible for the generation and regeneration of tissue. These processes are controlled by hormones and will generate new tissue rather than fat deposits, particularly when combined with a reduced calorie intake.

There are no special training programmes for losing weight. Similarly it is pure nonsense to suggest that increasing the number of repetitions and reducing the weights used in strength training will aid weight loss. We have no such thing as an "ideal weight" but merely a more favourable or less favourable composition. What counts is not what we weigh but whether that weight consists of muscle or fat.

Body composition is more important than body weight

A simple check

A simple way of checking how much fat you have is to measure a fold of skin near your navel. This can be done with a special clamp available from any medical supplies shop. For men 12 mm or less is considered normal. For women it is 15 mm. If it is much more you should reduce your calorie intake. However, it is essential to continue training.

If weight increases but skin-fold measurement remains the same this indicates an increase in muscle mass, something that is both safe and sensible.

However if weight drops without any reduction in skin-fold measurement this indicates a loss of muscle mass—not a good idea. If there is a reduction in both weight and skin-fold measurement this indicates a loss of fat. Assuming performance in training—your strength—remains the same it means you have retained muscle mass but if performance improves it means that your fat loss is greater than that shown on the scales because muscle mass has also increased.

To determine fat deposits measure a fold of skin near the navel

Do not check too often. Biological processes are rarely linear and tend to fluctuate in the short term. It is enough to check and record weight and skin-fold measurement monthly.

Relative versus absolute strength

A blue whale weighs some 140 tonnes and is 30 metres long. Although it is the largest and strongest animal on Earth it is, relatively speaking, the weakest as well. If stranded on land it suffocates because its own body mass compresses the lungs. In contrast, insects can carry many times their own body weight and jump over obstacles much larger than them. The absolute strength of an insect is low but its relative strength enormous. This law of nature can also be applied to man, albeit with minor variations. If you divide maximum strength output by body weight the resultant figure is something that can be classified as "relative strength". The higher it is the better.

What counts is the ratio of strength to body weight

Strength training for women

The principles of strength training apply equally to men and women. As already explained you cannot eliminate fat from specific areas. For women it is particularly important that they have a clear understanding of what can be changed because they are the main target of products that allegedly do this.

Cellulite

Cellulitis was the term used in the 1970s to describe the type of fat storage peculiar to women. With an "itis" ending it gave the impression that it was an illness or inflammation and advertisers were forced to change the term. It is now known as cellulite.

In the 1950s and as far back as the time of Rubens the female ideal was quite different from today. She had an ample figure with a full bosom. Both the sex idols of the 1950s and the models used by Rubens for his paintings had cellulite. On average these women were not more or less healthy than today. They were simply fatter.

The idea that cellulite can be eliminated by ointments is ridiculous as ointments cannot even penetrate the skin. In contrast strength training can help indirectly. Muscle tissue gets thicker and so the overlying skin is more taut.

Cellulite is not an illness but a form of fat storage peculiar to women

Firm not flabby

In fact women often achieve a rapid and spectacular improvement in their figure when they take up strength training. This may be due partly to the fact that untrained muscles make a person look fat even though they are not. They are simply flabby because muscle tone, that is, the "at rest" tension is too low. Training against resistance increases muscle volume following the increase in water content. This increases the osmotic pressure in the muscle cells that consolidate the tissue. In terms of physics it is the same process you see in a plant, which suddenly perks up after being watered. The effect is most evident in the larger muscles of the body such as the gluteals. However, training of pectoral muscles also has a positive effect on the bust. Although the breast has no muscles of its own and consists of glands covered with a liberal supply of fat, the breast will be lifted if the underlying muscles are strengthened. The state of our muscles is crucial to our external appearance—whether we are male or female. Everything sits where it ought to.

Good external appearance depends upon muscle condition

"Too much" muscle

The benefits of strength training for women are now well known. However, many women still fear it will make them look more masculine, that muscle mass will increase to the extent that is unattractive, at least in a woman. I can assure female readers that their fears are unjustified. As soon as you are happy with the way you look you merely "freeze" the load; continue to train regularly but do not increase the weight or number of repetitions. In this way you will remain "in shape" in all senses of the word throughout your life.

When you are happy with the way you look stop increasing the load

Old and strong

One day shortly after I started work as a trainer in the mid-1960s a 65-year-old turned up. He thought that strength training would do him good. He did not mind that most of the others were much younger. As a young man he had trained with weights at his gym and he well remembered how great he felt then. Nowadays he often felt tired and listless. He also assumed—and I want to emphasize this to all those over 50—that it was just because he was older!"

If you feel listless it is not the result of age

He started training and very soon achieved an amazing increase in muscle mass. His back stopped aching and his chronic fatigue was replaced by a feeling of alertness and an ability to concentrate throughout the day into the evening. He stood much more erect and had a spring in his step. "Like before" he said. A nice story. However, one day I saw him in Reception looking very sad. I asked him why he was not training today. He said he had a problem. He had enthused to his doctor about his new leisure pursuit. However, his doctor had told him to stop training. He had actually given him a "dressing-down" implying he had gone soft in the head. What was he thinking of starting something so stupid at his advanced age? Not only was he making a fool of himself, it was also bad for his health. It put too great a strain on the muscles, damaged the joints and harmed the back(!). The man was wondering whether the doctor might actually be right. After all, he would not advise against it without good reason, would he?

Strength training is not included in medical studies

I tried to encourage him saying that he should act on the basis of personal experience rather than that of another, even if that person were a doctor. I said he ought to overcome his doubts and continue training.

As the company grew I lost touch with him but I did hear that he continued training for many years. He may well have had feelings of guilt towards his doctor but that sometimes happens. The important thing was that he grasped the nettle and had the courage to disobey in his own interests. There are still many who lack the courage even today when strength training is largely accepted.

It is always said that we should "venerate old age". This idea appears not only in the Bible but many societies also have a cult of respect for the elderly. However, the idea actually comes from the elderly themselves: the old exploiting the young. Nowadays politicians talk about an alleged contract between generations. It does not exist. It is a lot of hot air. There is no reason to "venerate" the elderly. This contract between generations only exists in the minds of those who have become idle. We offer our seat to the elderly on the tube. We carry their luggage, help them on with their coats, open doors and so on. In seeking to minimize their load we actually enfeeble them. We kill them with kindness.

We kill the elderly with kindness

Fortunately there is evidence of a new trend. The average age of those doing strength training is increasing. Twenty years ago it was extremely unusual for older people to train regularly but now it is almost normal.

The importance of strength increases with age

Residents from a home for the elderly in Boston, all aged between 86 and 96 years, completed an 8-week programme in strength training. Exercises were restricted to the thigh muscles (quadriceps). The group recorded an average increase in strength of 174%. CT-scans showed that muscle mass had increased by 9% and walking speeds rose by 48%. Spectacular results, and for the residents a welcome improvement in their quality of life. However, it also begs the question as to what they had been doing previously, or more likely not doing previously that made such increases possible. There is a direct correlation between training potential and previous lack of exercise. If you are confined to bed for some time your training potential is enormous. This is because you regain strength at a faster rate.

Strength can be increased at any age

In principle if healthy there is no reason why the old should train differently from the young. The only thing to bear in mind is that the range of movement in some joints may well be much lower because of a lack of use for so long. This means they should work up to the full range of motion gradually. Special stretching exercises are not required. Just do the exercises on the machines correctly.

There is no reason why the old should train differently from the young

Theory and practice

From research we know that life started in a "primeval soup", the name given to the hot seas that existed at the dawn of history. Minute molecular organisms had the ability to multiply, producing first the single-cell organism and then the multiple-cell organism. The difference between multiple-cell and single-cell organisms was that some of the cells in the multiple-cell organisms performed certain specialist tasks. When combined these cells form organs and organ systems, for example, active and passive elements of the musculoskeletal system.

The cell is a fascinating organism. It is surrounded by a thin and partly permeable wall called a membrane, which provides protection. The cell maintains selective contact with its environment by giving off and absorbing matter. It exchanges heat, nutrients, oxygen, catabolic products and information with its external environment. In the primeval sea the fluid surrounding the cell was infinite. Human cells also live in a liquid environment. However, the volume of that liquid is less than the volume of the cell itself. The reason that the cell environment is not converted into a poisonous brew killing all life is due to the regulatory function performed by the blood supply. The body is constantly taking in water and nutrients and metabolic end products are eliminated through the bowels and the bladder. Such a "maintenance regime" requires specialized organs consisting of specialized cells.

What we are made of

All tissue types are interdependent

Tissue is the term used for a collection of cells, which form an organ or other body parts. There are various types of tissue. However, all are interdependent and life is only possible if they act in combination. There are six tissue types that we need to consider at this juncture: epithelial tissue, connective tissue, muscles, bones, nerves and blood.

Epithelium

This tissue is found only in multi-layer cell locations. It covers the external surface of the body (i.e., the skin) and lines hollow structures. Its role is to protect underlying tissue, absorb pressure and secrete.

Connective tissue

Connective tissue protects and supports. It pervades the entire body and consists primarily of inelastic collagenous fibre. Elastic connective tissue predominates only where connective tissue is subject to greater distortion. In the event of an injury, connective tissue acts as a repair substance. Nature is often overzealous in the good it does and creates an unnecessary amount of connective tissue, for instance, scars. Strong growth of connective tissue after an injury can restrict movements.

Ligaments link bones. Their structure is similar to tendons but have a higher percentage of elastic fibres, particularly the ligaments attaching to the rear of the spine.

The purpose of cartilage is to absorb pressure, for instance from a blow. Cartilage is elastic and so is found anywhere where distortion is essential. The ends of bone merge into cartilage. Intervertebral discs are an example of cartilage. Similarly the nasal bone terminates in a cartilage tip.

Tendons transfer muscle strength to the bones and are, therefore, subject to tension when muscles contract. They consist primarily of inelastic connective tissue. Most have a circular cross-section, but the tendons attached to abdominal muscles are flat and broad.

Connective tissue acts as repair material in the event of an injury

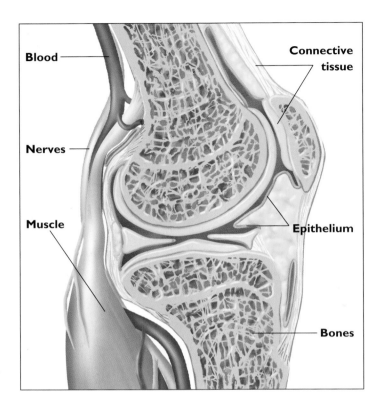

Muscles

Muscle fibres can be divided into three groups: smooth involuntary muscles, such as for digestive functions; striated voluntary muscles for skeletal movements and finally cardiac muscle, which is striated but involuntary. Our muscular system consists primarily of voluntary muscle fibres; in principle we can exert an influence on them. However, as organs they contain a significant percentage of connective tissue, blood vessels and nerves.

With the exception of the cardiac muscle all striated muscles are voluntary muscles

Bones

Bones are the hardest load-bearing tissue. Their stability comes from their salt content. Without salt a bone would be "decalcified" and would be flexible. Bones can soften if there is malnutrition, vitamin deficiency or a hormonal imbalance, for example rickets. A bone is a living organism. Strength training makes it stronger. Lack of tension weakens it.

Strength training also strengthens bones

Nerves

The nervous system is responsible for coordination and communication within the body. Nerves run through the body and like electricity cables can be of varying thickness. Compared with the speed at which electricity passes through a cable, nerve speeds are not that impressive: 50 to 120 metres per second. However, what is amazing is the number of cells. It is estimated that the grey matter of the brain contains some 150 billion cells. The smallest unit of tissue in the nervous system is the neurone. The smallest functional unit is the reflex arc.

The nervous system coordinates physical processes

Blood

Blood transports oxygen, carbon dioxide, nutrients, vitamins, hormones and catabolic products and performs a wide range of diverse functions. Each of us has about 5 litres of blood and if we lose more than 2 litres our life is threatened.

Blood transports metabolic and catabolic products

Activity and rest are mutually dependent

An organism is always in one of two states which are controlled by the central nervous system (CNS): sympathetic or parasympathetic. Sympathetic is the working state. When it is working the sympathetic division of our body's autonomic nervous system controls a whole range of processes. However they all have the same aim: to create with minimum delay a state of readiness for attack or flight. Blood moves from our internal organs to our muscles. Our digestive organs more or less stop work. The result is a "ready to fight" state.

Training should take place during the sympathetic phase. Overnight the body is in the recovery phase. This ends about 1 hour after breakfast, after which latent vitality increases. It drops somewhat about midday, rises again in the afternoon and drops to its lowest point at about midnight.

In a healthy organism the switch from work to recovery phase is well defined. A strong desire for food and rest will gain the upper hand. Blood flows back to the digestive system and adrenaline levels drop. This change of mode occurs largely without any action on our part. In fact we are not even conscious of it. In physiological terms one phase continues until the other automatically cuts in. However, this ideal state is now only present in animals and a few primitive people. It only rarely accords with modern life styles.

Malfunctions

The response of an organism to each phase depends upon its functional ability. If the response is ambiguous this is evidence of confusion in the central nervous system. Muscles remain in a state of semi-tension. We cannot perform (mentally or physically) to our full potential. At the same time we cannot "switch off" or relax. The causes are psychological, in particular a latent or acute anxiety that we cannot cope with everything we have to do (now called stress).

Any semi-tension not "extinguished" by work can cause damage to health in the long term. Merely asking someone who is stressed to relax makes little sense because one basic requirement is missing—genuine tension rather than imaginary tension. Genuine tension

Latent vitality fluctuates during the day

The switch from work to rest mode is automatic

is followed by relaxation and in this respect it is like breathing. We can only breathe out if we first breathe in. Relaxation is then an automatic response of the body and we do not have to worry about it.

Strength training demands high muscle tension. If deep sleep is one end of the scale then high muscle tension is the other. It is important to remember that the degree and intensity of the recovery phase is largely dependent on the previous working phase. If tension levels were high and brief, the resultant recovery will also be good. However, the reverse does not apply. You cannot store reserves of sleep to use later in a time of deficit. There is a tendency to postulate the reverse scenario. However, in reality the phrase "just relax" is an inner contradiction. The paradox is even greater in the expression "active relaxation". Only tension is "active". Relaxation is always passive, meaning it is only a reaction.

Tension is a prerequisite of relaxation

What does a muscle do?

A muscle contracts and in so doing moves bones at one or several joints. A muscle can only contract. It cannot extend itself. A muscle is extended by the contraction of its antagonist or by external pressure. To move a bone in the opposite direction the antagonist simply contracts—a simple principle of tension and counter-tension and the basis of the way we move.

Our musculoskeletal system works on the principle of tension and counter-tension

The term "origin" refers to the point where a muscle is secured to a normally less movable bone. The "point of attachment" is where a muscle attaches to a more movable part of the skeleton. Muscles can be one, two or multiple-joint muscles. This indicates how many joints the muscle covers and so moves. Depending upon the type of movement involved muscles can be in the same team—in which case they

During any given movement an antagonist can become a synergist

Theory and practice

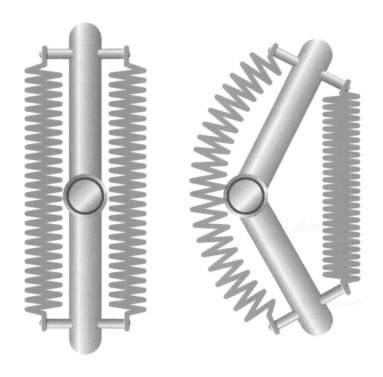

are known as synergist—or they can be in the opposite team, an antagonist.

The brain issues an order to the muscle to contract. The order runs through the spine to what is known as the motor endplate. The impulse can be either voluntary or involuntary. A stretch reflex is an involuntary impulse. When the doctor taps your tendon beneath the knee with a rubber hammer he is testing this reflex.

Where does a muscle get its energy when it contracts? A substance called adenosine triposphate (ATP) is stored in muscles, ready for immediate energy release. However, the supply is limited. ATP consists of three phosphate groups. When a muscle works one group precipitates out and this results in adenosine diphosphate (ADP). Another compound in the muscle, high-energy creatine phosphate, also breaks down when a muscle works, releasing one

The break-down of glycogen releases energy

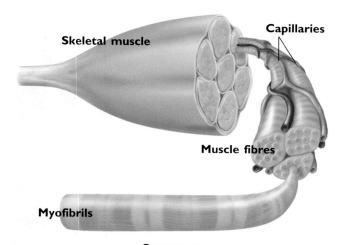

Skeletal muscle

Capillaries

Muscle fibres

Myofibrils

Sarcomere

Actin

Myosin

A-bands   I-bands

phosphate group. This combines with the ADP to form ATP and the muscle can continue working. However, after working for some 20 seconds the muscle can draw on another much greater source of energy: glycogen. As glycogen is broken down energy is released which in turn is used for the back formation of ATP and creatine phosphate. ATP and creatine phosphate are particularly important in strength training.

The longer a muscle works the more oxygen it needs. Oxygen is supplied through muscle capillaries. If the muscle works primarily without oxygen the work is termed anaerobic, whereas if more oxygen is used it is aerobic.

In practice the process of energy release is not as clear-cut as the theory would indicate. It is now assumed that the processes largely overlap. Very little

Muscles can work with or without oxygen

27

research has yet been done on the effect that these physiological processes have on the contraction of muscle fibres.

All or nothing

A muscle fibre works on the "all or nothing" principle. It either contracts or does not contract, there are no half measures. The central nervous system only calls on those fibres needed to achieve the necessary tension, with the rest coming along for the ride; they do not do any work. However, if the work continues for some time the working fibres start to tire. They drop out and the previously inactive fibres step in to continue the work. Eventually they also fatigue but are soon replaced. It is like a relay race except that it is actually a circle. Once the initial runners (fibres) have rested they return to work and continue their work of contracting the muscle and so it goes on.

In theory, if the resistance to be overcome is only slight, work can continue indefinitely because fibres have time to recover between shifts. However, once tension reaches a certain level, there are so many fibres actually working that there are too few waiting in the wings to take their place if effort is required for any length of time. As a result more leave than return. Each shift becomes shorter and shorter as fewer and fewer fibres have recovered sufficiently for a further shift.

So each ensuing cycle gets shorter and shorter as the nervous system desperately tries to locate fresh fibres until finally the muscle stops working. From then on movement is impossible.

The current theory on strength training is that the nervous system does not call up dormant fibres until these last few seconds or even fractions of a second. It is this process that triggers the increase in strength. Reserve fibres are muscles fibres that are not normally used. They are thin because they only contain a small

The nervous system only calls up the actual number of fibres required for a specific tension level

The nervous system only calls up reserve fibres shortly before a muscle stops working

amount of high-energy material. However, when called upon to work they respond by increasing in size and they then become active fibres. All training, apart from coordination training, is primarily about developing this unused energy potential. The significance of this is as follows:

The degree of muscle contraction during training is crucial in determining the success or otherwise of the training. The stimulus required by a muscle only occurs within a specific bandwidth. If the resistance is too low the existing active fibres can cope with the work and there is no need to recruit the dormant fibres. Training has no effect. On the other hand if tension is too high the muscle fatigues too quickly and the period under tension is too short. There is not enough time for the recruitment cycle to get going. The degree of tension and its duration are interdependent; it can be likened to shutter speed and aperture in photography, as one increases the other automatically decreases.

When exercising a muscle the first 10–20 seconds of an exercise can be regarded as a "warm-up". During this period the muscles use as many of the existing active fibres as possible, so creating the right environment for a training stimulus. Dormant fibres are not recruited until the final seconds of an exercise when almost all active fibres are exhausted. This is what makes training effective.

The first part of an exercise is a warm-up, that is, preparation for maximum effort during the final part

After a certain point, the amount of training, that is, the total period under tension, has a negative effect on training gain. The more extensive the training the more likely it will fail because tension will not reach the required stimulus threshold. This means that a system of training based solely on more training will have the reverse effect.

Heat makes you weaker

Articles in the popular press stress with monotonous regularity the importance of so-called warm-ups

Theory and practice

Diagrammatic representation of an untrained muscle (top) and a trained muscle (bottom). Active muscle fibres are thicker because they contain more liquid nutrients. Training converts the thin dormant fibres into active fibres. A muscle reaches its genetic potential when all dormant fibres have been converted into active ones.

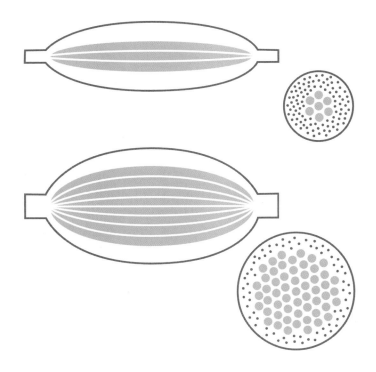

before any physical exertion and the potential risks if this is not done. Almost all these articles betray an amazing level of ignorance of the most basic laws of biology.

All too often the human body is likened to an engine, which has to be "warmed up" before it is put under load. The metaphor is not only inappropriate. It is wrong. Unlike an engine the body is a self-regenerating biological system. For example a steam engine or internal combustion engine are mechanical systems, which convert heat into mechanical energy. The more heat they produce the higher the resultant mechanical energy. In contrast, biological systems cannot convert heat into a different form of energy. They have to release it as it is superfluous and impedes performance. This is the basic difference between mechanical and biological systems.

A further difference is the temperature dependence of biological systems. Living organisms are extremely sensitive to temperature fluctuations, and the human body tries with all means at its disposal to maintain a constant temperature of 37 degrees Celsius. If the temperature in a muscle exceeds 43 degrees Celsius—that is only 6 degrees above normal—muscle protein starts to clot and death is instantaneous. In order to avoid such a disaster, the body cools its surface by sweating. That is why we sweat. Sweating does not "clean" the pores, it does not transport "waste-products" (there are none) and it does not eliminate toxins from the body. Similarly regular sweating (from a sauna or Turkish bath) does not affect the number of colds you get.

Heat reduces performance

More than 70% of muscle is water. Training increases the water content of muscles. If you lose water you lose much of your strength as well. Of course you can drink more to replenish the water but it is better to avoid the loss altogether.

Research has shown that enzymatic reactions double with every 10 degree rise in temperature. Although a slight increase in body temperature helps performance in the short term, the benefit soon disappears. In the case of strength training the benefit for the muscle to be trained only lasts a few seconds. Once body temperature reaches 39 degrees Celsius the use of oxygen in the muscle deteriorates dramatically and this soon leads to fatigue. Heat production is dependent upon body mass, the greater the body mass the quicker the temperature increase during activity. Women generally feel the cold more than men because they have less muscle mass.

The body is better equipped to deal with a drop in temperature: cold stimulates activity and blood is transferred from internal organs to the peripherals, that is, the muscles (sympathetic). We are all familiar with the invigorating effect of cold and the tiring effect of heat (para-sympathetic). As soon as our body senses it is getting too cold it starts to shiver. In order to shiver muscles have to work. This generates heat and body temperature is maintained.

There is no conclusive evidence to support the theory that warm-ups can reduce the risk of injury. This is not surprising because injuries, apart from those caused by external forces, have only one cause: jerky movements producing a load that exceeds the rupture limit of the tissue.

Warm-ups do not prevent injuries

Limbering up is useful

The situation is quite different with so-called limbering up. This is what athletes do before embarking on the complex series of movements required in competition. By doing a series of preparatory movements they retrieve stored images of the movements required for their sport. It is well known that muscle contractions have a reflex effect on mood. This means that limbering up is particularly useful as neurophysiological and mental preparation, but for strength training itself it is of no significance.

Limbering up is only of psychological and neurophysiological importance

Heat restricts muscle efficiency

What you can manage on an exercise bike is less than what you can manage on a bike outdoors. This is because the cooling effect of wind is absent inside. Heat does not improve performance. It reduces it. Even though this fact has been known for many years, it would appear that it has yet to penetrate the everyday world of training. Otherwise you would not find so many people on the fitness trail, in the gym, stadium or sports centre sweating profusely and overdressed. Even in summer they insist on doing a "warm-up session" despite being in a state of almost total collapse.

The ideal conditions for strength training are as follows:
- Maximum room temperature 20 degrees Celsius but preferably less
- Clothes that are loose and thin
- Warm-ups on a treadmill, exercise bike or other endurance machine are at best unnecessary. If they result in significant water loss (because room temperature too high or clothing inappropriate) warm-ups are counterproductive.
- Before doing anything that requires maximum effort, such as before an isometric test or a maximum number of repetitions, do a few contractions of the muscles to be tested.

Quantity and quality

More training does not necessarily mean better training. Training hard and long means maintaining a higher level of tension for longer. However, this is a contradiction in terms, in other words, a physiological impossibility. If you increase tension levels, the duration of that tension automatically drops and vice versa. For example if you can run 100 metres in 10 seconds there is no way that you can run 1000 metres in 10 × 10, that is 100 seconds. The intensity—the level of tension required for 100 metres—is only sustainable for 10 seconds.

More does not always help much

The argument that professional athletes can train all day is often used to explain the superiority of some sporting nations. Apart from the fact that most nations (or at least fans in those nations) use this argument to justify their own failures, it also displays a clear lack of understanding of the situation. A professional has just one advantage. Compared with an amateur who also has to work the professional has more time to recover. If an athlete were actually to train the entire

Theory and practice

Too much training weakens the immune system

day it would not be long before he or she had to stop. His performance would soon drop. In addition it would harm his immune system and so his general health would also deteriorate

By its very nature strength training is intensive. To a certain extent the volume of work is a necessary evil, which should be kept to a minimum. Each exercise requires a certain number of repetitions in order to activate biological processes in the muscle and the full programme multiplies this demand for energy. This is because you have to do a complete set of exercises to ensure that all skeletal muscles are subject to the required stimulus.

However, if training volumes exceed a certain level, the effect is reduced to zero or less than zero. If you increase training volumes the body has to make greater use of the reserves required to aid recovery after training. When preparing a training programme it is important to exercise the entire musculoskeletal system, but to achieve this with as few exercises as possible. What you should not do, as often happens, is literally to do every possible exercise in the repertoire.

The fact that some athletes train for several hours every day does not conflict with this theory. It merely indicates that they obviously have time to do this. However, it is safe to assume that they could achieve at least the same results with considerably less but more intensive training. I have met top athletes who have become world champions despite their training and not because it. If you have the right genetic makeup you will succeed despite what you do.

The misconception that "more" must equate with "better" is widespread not only in the sporting world but also in the minds of the general public: you only have to think of the innumerable cases of (medical) drug poisoning.

A good training programme has as few exercises as possible but as many as necessary

34

Progress — steady or in bursts

If we look at a graph showing the rate of increase in muscle strength most show a steep increase at the start of strength training followed by a levelling out. Why are we unable to maintain this initial rate of increase? Why does progress sometimes stagnate? Is it because we have achieved our strength potential or have we overtrained?

Instead of seeking an answer to these questions trainers have developed a strategy, which they hope will solve the problem. The magic formula is known as "periodization". It means alternating periods of low intensity but longer training with high intensity but shorter training. What this is designed to achieve remains a mystery!

In fact there is only one reason why progress stagnates and that is overtraining, always assuming of course that a muscle has not reached its genetic potential. Even many specialists are unaware of the fact that an athlete whose strength is increasing cannot cope with more training. He should be doing less. The ideal graph is one that shows a continuous and even increase from start to finish. A muscle can achieve its genetic potential in 18–24 months and after that it is merely a question of maintaining it.

The rate of increase tends to level out in time

Genetic potential is reached after training for 18–24 months

Muscle chains

When a muscle contracts it rotates bones around one or several joint axes. If the movement is a straight line this is achieved by a counter-rotation of at least two joints. For example when you stand from a squat, the femur rotates in the hip one way and the tibia rotates in the knee the other. The muscles used, in this case the gluteals and the quadriceps of the thigh, form a so-called muscle chain. This is the term for a group

A muscle chain is the term used for a group of muscles involved in a specific movement

Muscles have an influence not only on the joint they overlay but also on remoter parts of the body.

of muscles working together to perform specific movements. The example used above, standing from a squat, has actually been described in somewhat simplified terms. In reality each chain is made up of many muscles. For example a muscle not only exerts an influence on the joint over which its tendon stretches but also on more remote parts of the body. For example the gluteus maximus muscle, whose main role is to stretch the leg at the hip, "radiates" with its fibres to the latissimus dorsi muscle from where it exerts an influence on the elbow. The entire muscu-loskeletal system is, therefore, a closed, interdependent system.

The content of individual strength-training pro-grammes should take account of this relationship between individual muscles. If you strengthen legs and upper body but neglect the part in the middle, that

When you stand up from a squat your gluteals and quadriceps of the thigh form a muscle chain.

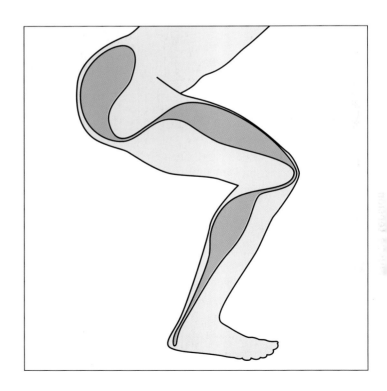

is, the location of the largest and most important muscles, you are storing up trouble for yourself. It means that your body has two strong parts connected by a weaker one. It is like having a strong door, a strong wall and thin hinges connecting the two. Such instances are not uncommon. Tests conducted by the University of Florida found that many of the participants, some of whom were extremely powerful athletes, had relatively weak back muscles.

You are creating a dangerous situation if your training neglects the middle part of your body

Strength curves

The strength of a muscle changes as it contracts. For example the strength of the biceps increases as it contracts. It exceeds the maximum when lower and

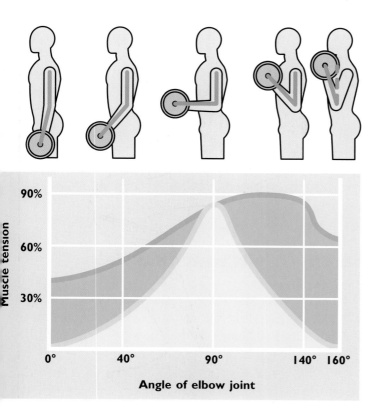

The lower curve shows the muscle tension during an exercise with a dumb-bell, the upper curve the tension required to train the entire length of the muscle.

Each joint function
has its own strength
curve

The greatest
potential for growth
lies in the final phase
of contraction

upper arm form a slight acute angle. After that strength declines sharply until the muscle is fully contracted. Consequently each joint function has its own strength curve different from that of other joints. There are both mechanical and physiological reasons for these differences.

In terms of training physiology a muscle cannot be regarded as a single unit. In reality an exercise will only increase strength in those joint positions where the load on the muscle exceeds the stimulus threshold. In other words our normal everyday activities influence strength curves and the result is "unnatural" strength curves. This means that strength curves vary from person to person with their shape depending upon the load on each muscle. As a general rule a muscle tends to be at its weakest in the final phase of contraction and so it is there that the greatest growth potential exists. This is because almost every load on a muscle—both at work and play—fails to reach this area.

Strength curves provide valuable information. For example a doctor treating a patient with back problems can use them to identify the precise point (angle) in a movement where the weakness occurs. If you "rectify" your strength curves you restore your musculoskeletal system to its proper state. However, you cannot achieve this with just "a little light exercise". You need special machines.

Strength without muscle?

Strength and muscle tissue do not develop in tandem. Whereas strength increases continuously muscle mass only increases in bursts. Based on a brief observation of the training process, many trainers started to wonder whether strength could be increased without increasing muscle mass. In fact this would be a biological "perpetuum mobile". Experts in the science of training were far too quick to believe in the high trainability of so-called intra-muscular coordination. It was thought that extremely high loads—up to 90–100% of maximum strength—could increase strength without increasing muscle mass, purely on a neuromuscular basis. Indeed there are studies that seem to show that strength can be increased without increasing muscle mass. However, a closer inspection of the test parameters reveals that there was no growth in either muscle mass or strength. This was because it was not strength that had improved but coordination of the musculoskeletal system as a whole. Individuals had not become stronger, just more skilful—"intermuscular" and not "intra-muscular" cooperation had improved

To measure muscle strength we need to isolate, as far as possible, the operation of individual muscles. This requires considerable technical effort and with many muscles is actually impossible. Most research into this subject is not worth the paper it is written on because the conditions required for accurate measurements are absent or incomplete. However, this is not to say that intra-muscular coordination, that is, making the most efficient use of muscle fibres within a muscle, does not exist. It does and although its potential is minimal it can be identified and as a sort of psychogram of a muscle it is of interest.

In terms of the options available to our body to meet demands imposed by its environment it will only give serious consideration to a development of muscle substance if it can find no other alternative. In this case our body is like a factory faced with a sudden influx of orders. It can solve the problem in several ways. It could recruit more staff but they need training and paying. Alternatively it could opt for the cheaper solution and rationalize production, improve coordination between individual processes and so increase

Improved intra-muscular coordination is often wrongly interpreted as increased strength

Intra-muscular coordination is rationalization in the muscle output at very little extra cost. If we regard muscle fibres as the "workers" and the muscle as the "factory", our body opts for the second model. Before recruiting "new" muscle fibres—which first need to be fed and coordinated—the central nervous system tries to improve the efficiency of existing fibres, that is, intra-muscular coordination. Only when it has exhausted this "cheaper" (in energy terms) option will it recruit new muscle fibres, that is new staff. Having recruited new fibres these new fibres gradually become more efficient. This in turn improves intra-muscular coordination and so even if demand continues to increase for several more weeks, further growth is not needed. However, if demand continues to rise beyond this period the process must be repeated. The hypothesis is self-evident: if demand increases muscles only grow tissue if they have exhausted all other reserves.

Strength is not increased until all other options are exhausted

Only one kind of strength

The strength of a muscle corresponds to the maximum possible tension that it can develop. In the world of training, different terms are used for different manifestations of strength. Static (isometric) strength is used to denote pure tension that triggers no movement. Dynamically concentric (positive) strength is where a muscle contracts and a resistance is overcome. Dynamically eccentric (negative) strength denotes "braking strength" which allows a slow extension of a muscle, for example, lowering the body slowly in "chins" or lowering a weight after lifting it. However, the difference between the three is merely the effect of internal friction.

Strength manifests itself in various forms

As the following test shows strength is the same irrespective of whether it is eccentric, concentric or static. The test involved the extensor muscle of the

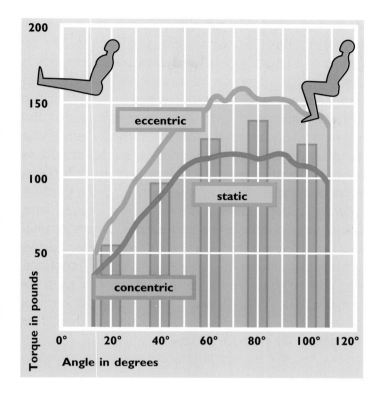

Torque in pounds

Angle in degrees

eccentric

static

concentric

The course of the strength curve is the same for all three types of load: static (bar chart), concentric (lower line) and eccentric (upper line). The overall strength only varies because the friction in the muscle varies.

lower leg, the quadriceps. A test machine was connected to a motor, which slowly rotated a lever arm to and fro at an angle of some 60 degrees. The test subject had to try and increase the speed of the lever arm on the upstroke and reduce it on the downstroke. The same muscles were, therefore, used in both cases and tension developed and maintained in identical muscles: firstly concentric (acceleration) and secondly eccentric (deceleration). A tensiometer was fitted to the lever arm to measure the pressure exerted. This pressure was displayed on a screen in the form of the graph, see below.

In the case of the concentric movement, muscles had to overcome both external resistance and internal friction. However, during the negative phase, that is, the eccentric movement, this friction helps as it acts as a brake. It took some of the load off the muscle

Friction makes a
concentric
movement more
difficult but makes
eccentric work
easier

so that eccentric strength looks the highest. This is why we can lower a heavier weight than we can lift. The static measurement, shown as a bar chart, is midway between negative and positive strength. This is because there was no movement and so there was no friction to make things easier or harder. As a muscle starts to fatigue friction increases and this is one reason why dynamic measurements are unreliable. Useable results (for scientific or medical purposes) can only be obtained from static tests.

Explosive strength is the ability to do a movement quickly and is dependent upon three factors, two of which can be changed:

- Strength (ie maximum strength),
- Coordination,
- Relative percentage of white fibres.

Training can improve strength. The practice of specific movement sequences can improve coordination. However, your dominant fibre type is determined by your genetic makeup.

Muscle stamina
increases in line with
strength

Stamina in the context of strength is the ability to maintain a specific muscle tension, either static or dynamic, for a specific period. Stamina increases in line with increases in maximum strength. For example when you first start training you may be able to do one chest-press repetition with 50 kg and six repetitions (about 60 seconds) with 40 kg (= 80%). After training for 6 months, you can do one repetition with 100 kg. Not only have you doubled your strength, you have increased your strength stamina by a similar ratio: you can now do six repetitions with 80 kg.

Training by the clock

Training by the clock is recommended because it has one major advantage over the conventional system of number of repetitions. It allows you to concentrate on doing the exercises properly and you cannot fool yourself. It works like this.

Start the exercise with the second hand at 12 o'clock. After that ignore the clock and concentrate on the relevant muscle. Simply try and continue for as long as possible. Do not try and do as many repetitions as possible as this will inevitably reduce the quality of the exercise and so reduce the effect.

Effort expended on maximum repetition is often at the expense of style

Always train slowly: 4 seconds for the contraction phase (raising the weight), hold the fully contracted position for 2 seconds and 4 seconds for the extension phase (lowering the weight). One complete repetition takes 10 seconds and so it takes about 1 minute to do six repetitions. However, this is a guide figure only. It is not the actual number of seconds that counts. What is important is to ensure that the exercise is done smoothly. You can do an exercise more slowly but not more quickly.

With a little practice you will find that you can start an exercise without waiting for the second hand to reach 12. Just look at your watch or the clock in the exercise room, make a mental note of the position of the second hand and start the next exercise. In this way you maintain training intensity because you minimize the gap between individual exercises. A stopwatch is not recommended because it is awkward to use and the temptation is to concentrate artificially on the exact number of seconds. The precise number of seconds is not important. Your aim is merely to identify whether you take longer or shorter than the time specified for the exercise. If longer, make a note to increase your training weight next time by 5–10%; if shorter, use the same weight next time. You should then record the time achieved.

When you first start training almost any resistance will do. However, it is a good idea to set yourself a specific time within which to achieve the required

After training for
some time you will
need to take account
of your genetic
muscle type

muscle tension. As you progress the duration of effective load starts to drop. Genetic differences become increasingly important and so training should gradually be geared to the dominant fibre type. Sixty percent of us can achieve the necessary stimulus in 60–90 seconds. Thirty percent of us have fast-twitch muscle fibres and tension is only required for 40–60 seconds. Only 10% of us are endurance types with predominantly slow-twitch fibres. In this case 90–120 seconds is required.

What does that mean for your training schedule? Initially, very little because the stimulus range of a muscle is still fairly broad. Only when strength has increased significantly will it be necessary to follow a more individual plan. The ideal time to change is when strength has remained static for several weeks.

One "set" or more?

The so-called stimulus threshold is exceeded when muscle tension reaches a certain level. The result is an increase in strength. However, if you exceed the threshold more than once during the same session, the result is not more growth but an unnecessary strain on the nervous system. Although this is something highlighted in considerable research dating back more than 30 years, almost all trainers still advocate so-called multiple sets. This is where the exercise is repeated several times. This is evidence of a basic misunderstanding, unfortunately by those who by the very nature of their work compound the resultant damage. Fortunately nature is tolerant and sometimes even benevolent. If you do an exercise properly you cannot repeat it immediately afterwards.

If you do an exercise
properly you cannot
repeat it

Correct order

If you trained just legs you would also notice a gradual increase in the strength of upper-body muscles. The effect would be less than if you had trained the upper body but it would be there all the same. However, this only happens with the larger muscle groups, the legs and the hips. Recent research has found considerably higher testosterone levels after simultaneous training of larger muscle groups with a high load time than after training of just the smaller muscles. This is the logic behind the theory that you should train larger muscles before the smaller ones:

Training of larger muscle groups also stimulates smaller muscles

- First exercise the gluteals, upper leg, abdominal and lower back muscles
- Then the upper back, pectoral and shoulders muscles, muscles of the upper arm, neck, lower leg and lower arm.

In terms of joints that means:

1. Hip joint
2. Knee joint
3. Lumbar spine
4. Shoulder joint
5. Cervical spine
6. Elbow joint
7. Ankle
8. Wrist

The order is particularly important if you want to train your heart muscle, that is, improve stamina. By training larger muscle groups first you quickly raise your pulse to an effective rate. Having raised your pulse rate, the subsequent exercises the less strenuous ones are sufficient to keep your pulse rate up until you have completed the exercises. Although it is useful to exercise larger muscles first and then smaller

Training larger muscle groups raises your pulse to an effective rate for training

ones, it is not essential. It depends upon your objectives—therapy or rehabilitation—and a different order may be preferable.

Single- and multiple-joint exercises

There are some 40 exercises in all not including the variations. For example, with the leg press the upper body can be in one of three angles. By changing the angle you can slightly change the main focus of the load within the muscle chain. Similarly, with a lateral raise you can vary the angle of the lower arm. These subtle differences are mainly relevant when a machine is used for therapy purposes and so there is no need to consider them here.

Basically there are two different types of exercises: single-joint and multiple-joint exercises. Single-joint exercises are ideal for correcting strength curves because the tension is correct throughout the range of motion. However, each exercise only trains a few muscles and this limits its spread. In contrast multiple-joint exercises train all muscles in a chain simultaneously. However, with most multiple-joint exercises the tension is only correct in two-thirds of the range of motion. This is because multiple-joint exercises exert pressure more or less in a straight line, which means that unlike single-joint exercises resistance is not applied direct. For example when straightening the leg at the knee in the leg press you would need a resistance in excess of 1 tonne if the load on the quadriceps in this position were to correspond to its strength curve and this would exceed the fracture load of the bone. A range of motion of two-thirds is still very good compared with bending the knees with dumb-bells. In this case only one-fifth of the movement is above the threshold level. Single-joint

A slight change in the main load point is only important for therapy purposes

Only with single-joint exercises is the tension precise throughout the movement

exercises are recommended for beginners because most have strength curves distorted by the stresses and strains of everyday life and sport.

Technology

Nobody has yet written a historical analysis of strength training

There is a history of body culture and more narrowly a history of sport. Training has tended to play a somewhat minor role because cultural and social issues have been dominant. Nobody has yet completed a historical analysis of training and equipment.

History of strength training

Murals from Ancient Egypt (3000 BC) depict men and women doing strength training. The first recorded training manual was written about 1400 BC. Written in Hittite cuneiform script it was found in the Palace at Boghazköy, at that time the capital of the Hittite Empire in the northern part of Central Anatolia. The manual, which is extremely detailed, describes the training required for chariot racing. Similarly the Chou Dynasty (1122–249 BC) in China seems to have been familiar with strength training. The test to join the army consisted of lifting heavy weights. It is thought that Confucius (551–479 BC) trained with weights of incremental size.

The principle of training with incremental weights dates back more than 3000 years

The Greek Milon of Kroton (500 BC), a friend of Pythagoras, did strength training by lifting a young bullock every day. As the bullock grew heavier and heavier Milon grew stronger and stronger. Milon was Olympic wrestling champion continuously from 532–516 BC. Galen of Pergamon (129–199 AD), the physician to the gladiators and later to personal physician to the Roman Emperor Marc Aurel, considered physical training a part of medicine.

Barbells made from dressed stone were used in Southern Asia as early as the fist century AD. Each stone remained in use over several generations. Each was inscribed with the name of the owner and was subsequently handed down to the next generation.

The Romans institutionalized physical training with their thermal baths. We know that the gladiators fighting in the Colosseum in Rome were very muscular and "sexually alluring". They had their own training centres on the outskirts of Rome where they prepared for fights. Surprisingly we have little evidence of their actual training but the bodies depicted in contemporary sculptures leave us in no doubt that they were developed by some form of systematic training.

With the fall of the Roman Empire Christian fanatics gained the upper hand and destroyed what there was of pagan cultural heritage. They were more interested in the hereafter. This explains the general contempt with which the body and sensuality in general was regarded during the Middle Ages.

It was not until the Period of Enlightenment that the body gradually shed its bad reputation as the vessel of sin. In 1816, Friedrich Ludwig Jahn (1778–1852) published a study of the methodology of physical training. In his work *Die deutsche Turnkunst* [German Gymnastics] he describes in detail the exercises done at the time. His instructions on how to do chins show that Jahn was aware of the importance of isolating the muscles to be trained. "In this exercise arms do all the work to raise the body and so the legs and the rest of the body must be kept as still as possible".

From the mid-19th to the start of the 20th century strong men performed tricks in music halls. To make it more exciting prizes were offered to anyone who could perform the same tricks. Although muscle strength was a requirement it was not crucial to success. Some of these acts of strength were extremely complex and demanded a high level of skill. Each strongman had a specific routine. There was none of the standardization that is characteristic of sport today.

Eugen Sandow (1867–1925)—real name Karl Friederich Müller—was probably the most famous strongman of modern times. He was the first who not only wanted to impress others with his physical feats but was also interested in his overall physique and can be considered as the inventor of bodybuilding. He enjoyed considerable fame in the United States for his body and was even regarded with enthusiasm by intellectuals of the time. Sir Arthur Conan Doyle (1859–1930), the English writer and creator of Sherlock Holmes, thought "his achievements outranked almost all others in his generation". Charles Atlas (1892–1972), one of the last supermen of that era, ran distance-learning courses selling more than 3,000,000 courses in total.

The 20th century saw the rise of institutionalized sport and the sports industry. Strongmen were assigned to history.

Stages in the development of training

The history of training equipment can be divided into four stages.

Callisthenics

Free exercises are those that require no equipment or only that required for performance purposes. Their aim is to conjure up an image. They are an expression. They are designed to impress, that is their purpose: leaping into the air from a squat (to frighten the enemy), jumping, throwing, gestures indicating subjugation, submission or combat, all of which can be found in dance rituals, ballet, military parades, group gymnastics, aerobics and ceremonies of all types. Although directed primarily at an audience, free exercises also increase the performance capabilities of the individual. They improve our ability to overcome gravity.

Resistance exercises

The next stage was the deliberate use of an external resistance, such as a stone, tree or living being. Even at that time it was recognized that the use of a resistance builds strength. The purpose was training rather than just performance.

Exercises using a progressive resistance

The next stage was to achieve an incremental increase in the load by selecting or manufacturing equipment with a range of weights or degrees of difficulty. The first barbells of this new era were two cannon balls joined by an iron bar. The weight of cannon balls varied which allowed the production of barbells of differing weights. However this method of training required a large number of barbells, both light and heavy. Consequently the development of barbells with discs was a major advance. By adding or removing a disc from the barbells you could quickly change the total weight.

The development of barbells with discs allowed for a quick adjustment of the load

Exercises with a variable resistance

The first "pure" training machines were developed by Dr Max Herz at the end of the 19th century. He designed and produced machines for physiotherapy, which incorporated a resistance that changed in the course of the exercise. The change in resistance mirrored the change in the strength of the user during the exercise. Herz realized that strength only increased in those joint positions subject to a load above the stimulus threshold. However, if joints are to function properly strength must be developed throughout the entire range of motion. Herz calculated the ideal strength curve for each joint in the

Dr Herz was the first to develop machines where the resistance changed during the exercise

The development of the pullover machine made it possible to exercise the entire *latissimus dorsi*

The Nautilus range developed by Arthur Jones represented a new standard in the design of training equipment

human body. He then designed a mechanical component that would replicate this strength curve, an eccentric wheel (cam) that set the torque required to move a lever in the various joint positions. Herz supplied his equipment to many clinics but in the ensuing turmoil and disasters of two World Wars his idea was unfortunately lost.

In 1972 the inventor and entrepreneur Arthur Jones developed a training machine which—even though Jones had never heard of him—incorporated Herz's idea. Jones, who now lives in Florida, developed a "pullover" machine, which isolated and exercised the *latissimus dorsi*. Unlike previous exercises for this muscle (chins, pull devices, rowing exercises) the pullover machine applied resistance direct to the humerus, the bone moved by the *latissimus dorsi*. For the first time it was possible to isolate this important muscle and exercise it without involving closer but weaker muscles (the biceps). Under the name "Nautilus" Jones developed 40 machines based on the same principle and covering most movements in the human body. Within a few years his company was a market leader in training equipment. It is thanks to Arthur Jones that the concept of a changing resistance was established as a development stage in its own right. This was is not to say that the principle was understood by all. Undoubtedly one reason for his success was the innovative design of the machines. They were quite different from previous devices, intended to solve specific biomechanical problems.

With his machine for the lower back muscles (lumbar extensors) Jones managed to penetrate the medical profession. This machine isolated, tested and trained these muscles. Jones sold the Nautilus company and set up the MedX Corporation. He then devoted many years to back problems and the benefits that training can provide. However, he also realized that he could improve his earlier Nautilus machines. So in addition to MedX test and therapy machines, used solely for medical purposes, he designed a range of machines to exercise other muscles.

How a cam works

The Herz machines and those developed 50 years later by Jones created a resistance that changes as the movement progresses. This was achieved by a cam and the way it works is shown in the diagram below.

The lever arm rotates in the direction of the arrow and provides a connection between A and O. The cam is permanently fixed to the lever arm. The complete unit can be rotated around the axis O.

For the sake of simplicity the cam on the diagram describes a spiral curve. In reality the curve described by the cam varies depending upon the muscle whose load it is designed to regulate. The cam is fixed to a tension strap at point 'a'. At the other end of the strap is a weight Q. The level of tension exerted on the

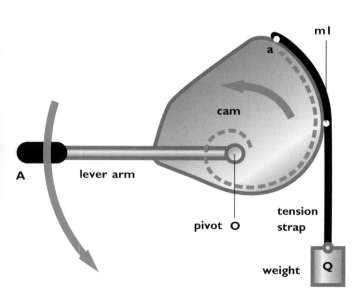

The cam allows the resistance to change continuously: the force required to move the weight is infinitely variable because the shape of the cam is irregular.

In most cases the cam plots an exponential curve

lever arm by the weight Q depends upon the distance horizontally between point 'm1' and the axis O. The closer it is to the axis the less the tension. If a circular disc were connected to the lever arm instead of an eccentric one the tension would remain the same irrespective of the position. The cam technology is not required on all machines because with most multiple-joint machines the load can be varied during the exercise by a simpler mechanism.

What critics say about machine-based training

Machine-based training has become increasingly popular. Machines are replacing dumb-bells. Despite this they still have their vocal opponents. Those who advocate training with "free weights", such as dumb-bells, use the following arguments.

'Barbells allow greater freedom of movement'

With a machine the course of a movement is dictated by physiological needs

False, in fact the opposite is true. Gravity dictates the precise course of a movement with a barbell. If you doubt this, try bench-press exercises lifting a barbell along a plane other than one vertical to the Earth's axis. Machines also dictate the course of the movement. However, in this case the movement does not necessarily follow gravity, rather it corresponds to the physiological needs of the muscle.

'Barbells also work those muscles not directly involved'

True, they do work these muscles but the load is below the stimulus threshold; training tires them but the stimulus is absent. To reach the required stimulus threshold you must exercise individual muscles directly.

'Barbells are better for athletes than machines because they also improve coordination'

True but only the coordination required for the specific exercise, as coordination skills are not transferable. Replicating movements required in a sport but under more difficult conditions is probably the commonest form of stupidity found in sports training. The real reason for the popularity of barbells is an emotional one. You can only use the coordination developed with barbells if you are a weight or power lifter. They are the only disciplines that require training with heavy barbells, as they require the coordination that comes from lifting them. The origin of barbells is a pointer in this respect. They were originally used as aids in strength demonstrations at funfairs and circuses as they were better than any other equipment when it came to lifting very heavy weights. In other words barbells can train strength and "demonstrate" it as well. The aim is to see what you can achieve and to show others as well.

Strength training is not intended to improve coordination

Barbells were not originally intended for training

The advantages of strength machines

The five main benefits of training with machines rather than free weights or exercises using your own body weight are as follows:

1 Accurate control of the tension through the entire range of motion, it is not random. The muscle exceeds its stimulus threshold throughout its range, from full extension to full contraction. This prevents or corrects intra-muscular imbalance.

2 It guides (two-dimensional) movements. "Incorrect" movements are (almost) impossible reducing the risk of injury to near zero.

Technology

Physiological tension throughout range of motion, no risk of injury, maximum muscle isolation, productive training from the start and an exact measurement of progress are the advantages of machine-based training

3 The pad, supports and restraints, which form part of the machine, ensure that individual muscles are isolated. This facilitates cross-sectional stimuli.

4 Machine training does not require coordination skills. You do not have to "learn" and so training is productive from the start.

5 The gain with machine-based training is pure strength; the gain is not a mixture of strength and coordination.

The main difference between the various makes of machine is their ability (or inability) to deal with these five points. That is not to say that strength machines cannot cause problems. There can be technical, space, investment or educational problems. In the final analysis it all comes down to cost.

Friction is a technical problem inherent with any training machine. For example: a biceps exercise on a poorly maintained biceps machine with a weight of 50 kg. As you lift the weight (contracting the biceps) you have to overcome 50 kg plus 20% due to friction: 60 kg. However, when the weight is lowered resistance drops from 60 kg to 40 kg. In terms of training physiology the load during the extension phase is inadequate and so a waste of time. In other words at the very point where resistance should be as high as possible (see page 40 "Only one kind of strength") friction in the machine reduces resistance further. Features designed to minimize friction levels greatly influence the cost of a machine: ball bearings rather than bearing bushes, bars rather than chains or V belts, a large weight stack to minimize both the required stroke ("reduction ratio") and initial friction, guide bars made of polished steel, bushings made from porous bronze, etc. MedX machines have even dispensed

Friction is minimized on quality machines

with guide bars. However, this means that the weight of the weight stack is twice that of comparable machines because the path of the weight during the exercise must be 50% shorter.

What the future holds

Groundbreaking progress such as that described above is a rarity. It is not enough to invent something "new". The time has to be right as well. Jones first started production of his pullover machine in 1948 but there was no interest. Demand did not develop until 1968 when the fitness boom started.

So what developments are likely in the future? The next development, the fifth stage, could well be machines that train several muscles—muscle chains—at once whilst still maintaining the benefits of existing machines:

- progressive resistance,
- adequate change in resistance during exercise,
- direct resistance (not "filtered" through weaker muscles).

Such machines represent the future. Anyone closely involved with the human musculoskeletal system knows that even today's best machines are still a long way from being perfect. The design of a perfect machine for the biceps, at first glance a fairly simple muscle, is a technical and mathematical nightmare. To ensure the correct load, from full extension to full contraction of the biceps, you need to integrate a minimum of three strength curves, each of which affects the other two. "Correct" contraction of the biceps starts with hands in the so-called pronate position with arms extended backwards and ends with hands in the supinate position behind the head. Try to maintain tension in the biceps during the entire

Effective machines that combine several locomotor functions are still a long way off

57

movement, including the final position when your arms are behind your head. In this position you will experience a spasm in the biceps indicating that you have contracted the maximum possible number of fibres.

If a machine could be developed that subjected major muscle groups to this form of load, it would significantly reduce training times and maximize results. It would also exercise many muscles simultaneously making it ideal for cardiovascular training.

If strength training were to become an integral part of our hygiene routines, we could solve problems not currently even associated with strength problems. However, we have not yet reached this stage. The standard of (professional) equipment currently available varies depending upon the skills of manufacturers or their advisers.

Muscles

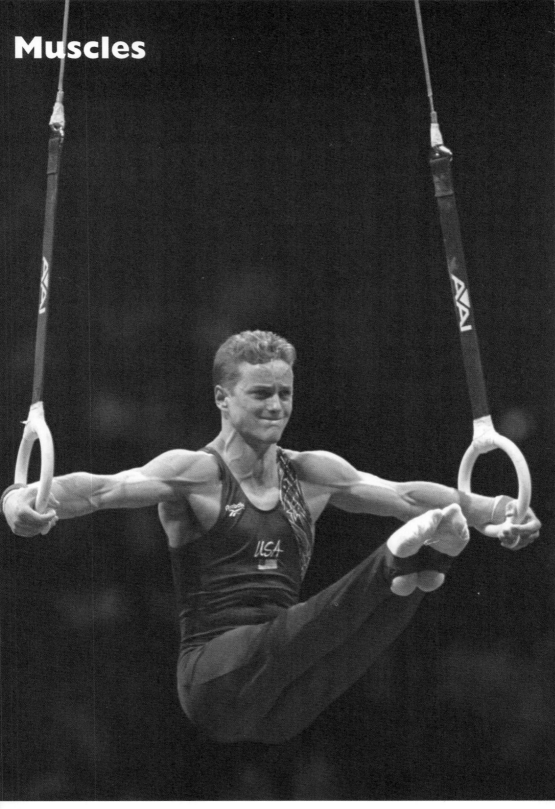

John Macready at the US Gymnastics Olympics trials, Boston, Massachusetts, 1996 (by courtesy of Allsport: photograph by Doug Pensinger).

Trunk muscles

	Muscle	Function	Exercises	Origin & insertion
1	**Deltoid muscle, front section** *m. deltoideus – pars clavicularis*	Raises arm forwards	**D6**	**Origin:** outer end of clavicle, shoulder level & spine of scapula **Insertion:** humerus
2	**middle section** *m. deltoideus – pars acromialis*	Raises arm sideways	**E2** **E1**	
3	**Greater pectoral muscle (m. pectoralis major)**	Moves arm forwards and inwards and shoulder girdle forwards	**D5** **D6** **D7** **E3** **J4**	**Origin:** clavicle, sternum, sheath of straight muscle of the abdomen **Insertion:** humerus
4	**Serratus anterior muscle**	Pulls shoulder blade forward allowing you to raise arm above the horizontal	**E1** **E3**	**Origin:** ribs 1–9 **Insertion:** medial edge of shoulder blade, upper and lower angle of scapula
5	**Straight muscle of abdomen (m. rectus abdominis)**	Brings thorax closer to pelvis	**A2** **F2**	**Origin:** costal cartilage 5–7, xiphoid process of sternum **Insertion:** pubic bone
6	**Oblique muscle of abdomen (m. obliquus abdominis)**	Allows you to bend to side and rotate trunk	**F1** **J9**	**Origin:** outer surface of ribs 5–12 **Insertion:** iliac crest, inguinal ligament, pubic tubercle, "linea alba"
7	**Sternocleido-mastoid muscle**	Bends head and cervical spine sideways	**G3**	**Origin:** sternum and clavicle **Insertion:** mastoid process and upper nuchal line
8	**Trapezium muscle, upper section** *m. trapezius pars descendens*	Raises shoulder blade. Tilts head to side and back	**G1** **G3** **G5**	**Origin:** squamous part of the occipital bone, spinal processes of cervical & thoracic vertebrae
9	**central section** *m. trapezius pars transversa*	Brings shoulder blade closer to spine, holds shoulder blade in place	**C5** **C7**	**Insertion:** clavicle, shoulder level, spine of the scapula
10	**lower section** *m. trapezius pars ascendens*	Lowers shoulder blade	**C3 J2** **J3 D7** **J4**	

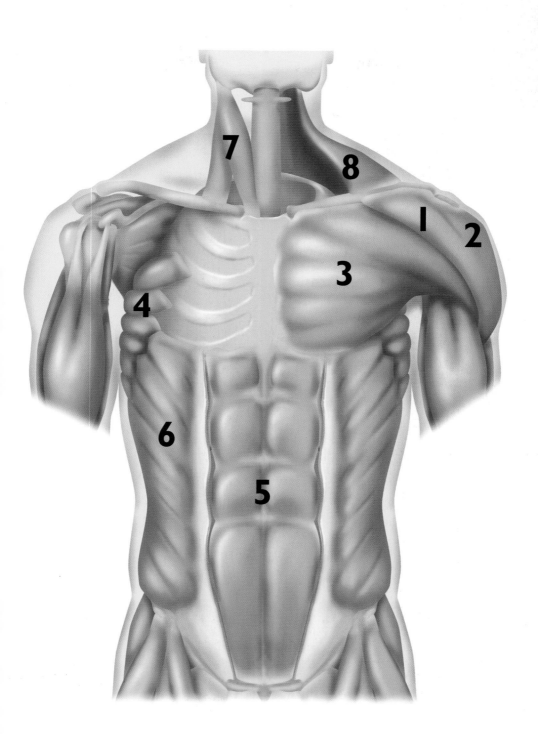

Muscles

	Muscle	Function	Exercises	Origin & insertion
11	**Deltoid muscle, rear section** *m. deltoideus pars spinalis*	Moves arm horizontally to rear	**C5**	**Origin:** outer end of clavicle, shoulder level and spine of the scapula **Insertion:** humerus
12	**Latissimus dorsi muscle** (*m. latissimus dorsi*)	With arm above head pulls it down and back	**C1** **C3** **C7** **J2** **J3**	**Origin:** spinal processes of lower six thoracic vertebrae, all lumbar vertebrae, sacrum and iliac crest **Insertion:** intertubercular groove of humerus
13	**Erector muscle of the spine** (*m. erector spinae*)	Holds spine erect	**A1** **F3** **G5**	**Origin:** transverse processes of all vertebrae, sacrum, iliac crest **Insertion:** transverse processes of cervical, thoracic and lumbar vertebrae
14	**Teres major muscle (*m. teres major*)**	Brings arm closer to trunk with a slight internal rotation and the upper arm backwards	**C1 C3** **J2 J3** **C5 C7** **E4**	**Origin:** lower third of shoulder blade **Insertion:** intertubercular groove of humerus
15	**Teres minor muscle (*m. teres minor*)**	Rotates arm outwards around its longitudinal axis and pulls arm backwards	**C5** **E5**	**Origin:** lower third of shoulder blade **Insertion:** greater tubercle on humerus
16	**Rhomboid muscle (*m. rhomboideus*)**	Pulls shoulder blade up and back towards spine	**C5** **C7**	**Origin:** spinal processes of the lower cervical and upper thoracic vertebrae **Insertion:** central margin of shoulder blade
17	**Superior and inferior oblique muscles of head** (*m. obliquus capitis* **superior** and *m. obliquus capitis* **inferior**)	Extends head backwards and rotates it	**G5**	**Origin:** atlas, axis **Insertion:** back of head, atlas
18	**Greater and lesser posterior straight muscle of head (*m. rectus capitis posterior* major and minor)**	Extends head backwards and rotates it	**G5**	**Origin:** atlas and axis **Insertion:** base of the skull

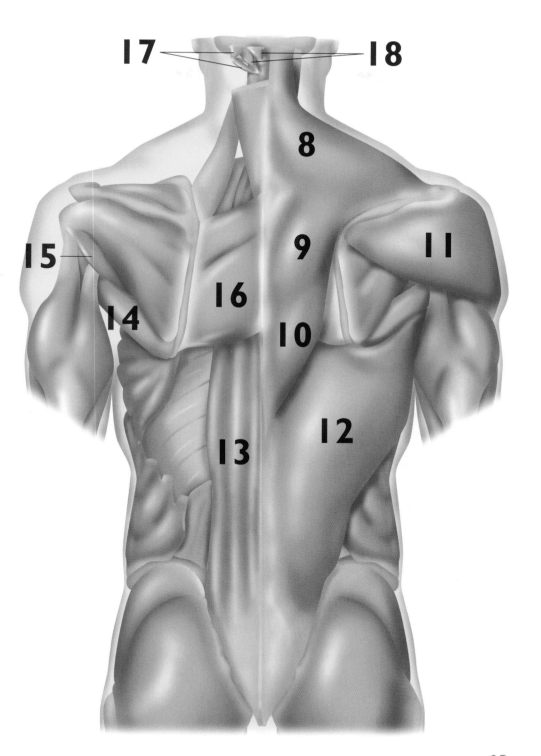

Leg muscles

	Muscle	Function	Exercises	Origin & insertion
1	**Iliopsoas muscle (*m. iliopsoas*)**	Raises thigh forwards and upwards	**A2**	**Origin:** lowest thoracic vertebrae and lumbar vertebrae 1–4, ala of ilium **Insertion:** femur
2	**Quadriceps muscle of thigh (*m. quadriceps femoris*)**	Stretches leg at knee joint	**B1** **B6**	**Origin:** iliac spine, acetabulum, anterior and lateral surface of femur **Insertion:** tibia
3	**Thigh adductors (*m. adductores*)**	Pulls leg towards central line of body	**A4**	**Origin:** ischium and pubis **Insertion:** femur
4	**Sartorius muscle**	Rotates upper leg outwards and lower leg inwards	**A3**	**Origin:** anterior upper iliac spine (pelvis) **Insertion:** tibia
5	**Anterior tibial muscle (*m. tibialis anterior*)**	Raises foot at ankle	**B8**	**Origin:** anterior surface of tibia **Insertion:** metatarsal bones
6	**Long extensor muscle of the toes**	Extends toes	**B8**	**Origin:** tibia, fibula **Insertion:** toe bones
7	**Greatest gluteus muscle (*m. glutaeus maximus*)**	Extends leg at hip joint	**A1** **B6**	**Origin:** ilium, sacrum and coccyx **Insertion:** femur, femoral fascia
8	**Biceps muscle of thigh (*m. biceps femoris*)**	Bends leg at knee joint and extends leg at hip joint	**A1** **B5** **B6** **B7**	**Origin:** ischial tuberosity, dorsal aspect of femur **Insertion:** head of fibula
9	**Semitendinous muscle**	Bends leg at knee joint and extends leg at hip joint	**A1** **B5** **B6** **B7**	**Origin:** ischial tuberosity **Insertion:** tibia
10	**Gastrocnemius muscle**	Lowers foot at ankle	**J1**	**Origin:** femur **Insertion:** calcaneous tuberosity
11	**Soleus muscle**	Supports Gastrocnemius muscle	**J1**	**Origin:** fibula and tibia **Insertion:** calcaneous tuberosity

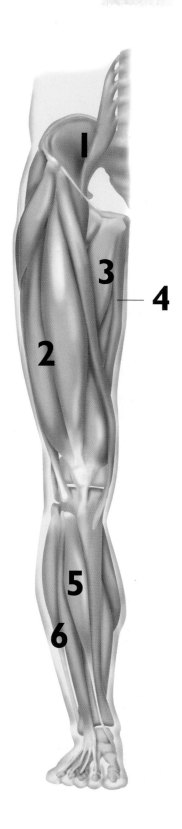

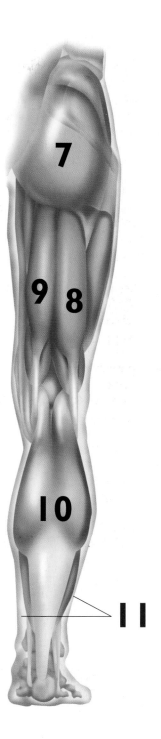

Arm muscles

	Muscle	Function	Exercises	Origin & insertion
1	**Biceps muscle of arm (*m. biceps brachii*)**	Bends (together with two smaller flexors not visible on illustration) arm at elbow, rotates forearm outwards	**C3 J2 J3 C7 H1 H4**	**Origin:** superior glenoid tuberosity of scapula, coracoid process **Insertion:** radius
2	**Triceps muscle of arm (*m. triceps brachii*)**	Stretches arm at the elbow and pulls upper arm backwards	**D6 J4 D7 J5 E1 E3 H2**	**Origin:** inferior glenoid tuberosity of scapula, humerus **Insertion:** olecranon
3	**Hand and finger flexors (*mm. flexores carpi*)**	Bends fingers and hand inwards	**H5**	**Origin:** humerus **Insertion:** metacarpal bones
4	**Hand and finger extensors (*mm. extensores carpi*)**	Extends fingers and hand outwards	**H6**	**Origin:** humerus **Insertion:** metacarpal bones, rear tendon sheath of fingers

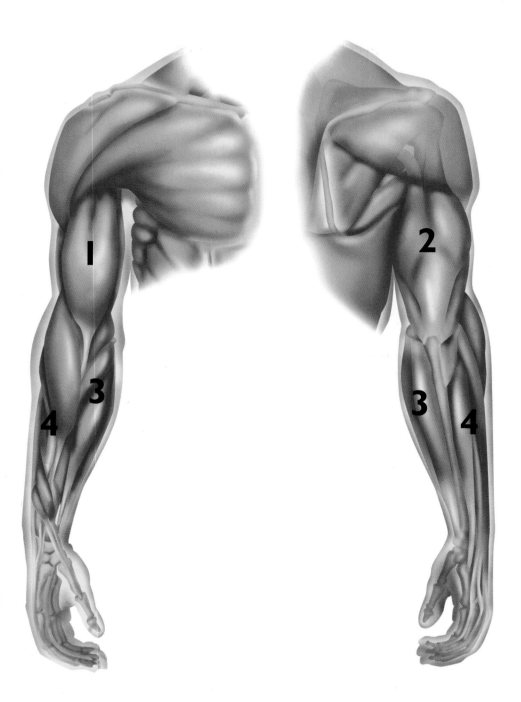

Training principles

The following training principles are theory translated into practice. In the absence of any particular disability or illness they should be followed.

If you have problems with your musculoskeletal system or your general health consult a doctor qualified in medical strengthening therapy wherever possible. Doctors, including sports injury specialists, without this additional training cannot identify possible risks because they are unfamiliar with the nature of the training. However, doctors trained in medical strengthening therapy are familiar with the exercises and their effect, allowing them to devise training programmes tailored to your needs.

Lack of patience and anxiety are the main reasons for ignoring the training principles. Be under no illusion, training reveals your inner state of mind. It impels you to focus on your inner self and this in itself is beneficial. You may find there are times when you have to force yourself to train although you do not want to or are too busy with "other things".

Be honest with yourself. Do not try and impress yourself or anyone else with your own prowess. For productive training a strong will is less important than the need to do the exercises carefully.

Observe the following Training Principles at all times.

1 Train once or twice a week. Each session should cover the entire body.

2 Do a maximum of 10 exercises per session. When you have doubled your strength reduce the number of exercises to 8. When you have trebled it reduce the number to 6.

3 Train the muscles of the lower body first.

Doctors qualified in medical strengthening therapy can identify possible risks associated with training

Strength training forces you to focus on your inner self

Be honest with yourself

4 Select a weight that allows you to do an exercise for 60–90 seconds. Do 6–9 repetitions. The positive movement—raising the weight—should take at least 4 seconds. The negative phase—lowering the weight—should also take 4 seconds. In between, as the muscle is fully contracted, maintain tension for 2 seconds.

5 At all costs avoid sudden "explosive" movements. They are dangerous and counterproductive.

6 Only do each exercise to the point of local fatigue, that is, until you can no longer do a complete movement. If you can do the exercise for longer than 90 seconds make a note to increase the weight about 5% next time.

7 Avoid any "help": do not turn, wriggle or swing the body. Isolate the relevant muscles as far as possible.

8 Relax muscles not used in the exercise. In particular relax the hand, neck and facial muscles.

9 Do not hold your breath during the exercise but breathe in as required. The rhythm of breathing does not necessarily have to coincide with the rhythm of the exercise.

10 Wherever possible keep the interval between individual machines to a maximum of 15 seconds as this allows your heart and circulation to benefit as well.

11 Do not do more than one set of exercises on each machine. Two consecutive sets do not increase the stimulus.

12 Do not increase the weight if this reduces exercise quality.

13 At the end of each session enter weight for the next session on your training card.

Training principles

14 Drink water (without additives) before, during and after training.

15 Leave a gap of at least 48 hours between each training session

Exercises

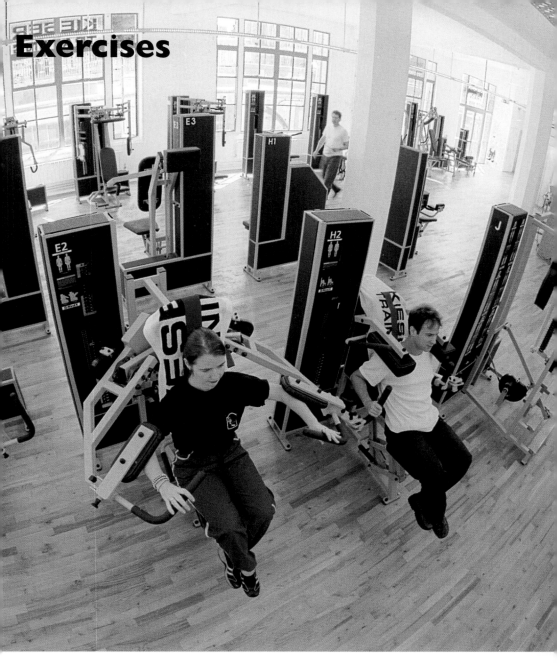

Photograph by Mark Hakansson, London.

Exercises

List of exercises

There are currently a total of 41 exercises, 10 of which are selected for any given training programme. Exercises are divided into categories A–H with each letter covering a specific part of the body. Exercises with a "J" designation are done on a multi-function machine: they exercise a range of muscles. Where there is a gap in the number designation, (B2, B3 and B4) it is reserved for machines that have not yet been developed. The graphic depictions of muscles involved in an exercise on the following pages only show the prime movers.

Note: the graphic depiction of muscles involved in an exercise on the following pages only show the prime movers.

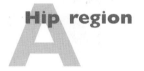

Hip region

A1	Hip extension
A2	Torso flexion
A3	Abductor
A4	Adductor

Legs

B1	Leg extension
B5	Prone leg curl
B6	Leg press
B7	Seated leg curl
B8	Tibia dorsiflexion

Back

C1	Pullover
C3	Torso arm
C5	Rowing torso
C7	Row

D5	Arm cross
D6	Chest press
D7	Seated dip

Chest

E1	Neck press
E2	Lateral raise
E3	Overhead press
E4	Internal rotation – shoulder
E5	External rotation – shoulder

Shoulders

F1	Rotary torso
F2	Abdominal
F3	Lower back

Trunk

G1	Neck & shoulder
G3	4-way neck – side
G4	4-way neck – front
G5	4-way neck – rear

Neck

H1	Biceps
H2	Triceps
H3	Wrist pronation
H4	Wrist supination
H5	Wrist curl
H6	Reverse wrist curl
H7	Hand grip

Arms

J1	Calf raise
J2	Front chin
J3	Parallel chin
J4	Dip
J5	Triceps extension
J9	Side bend

Multi-functional

Hip extension

Select weight. Lie on your side facing the weight stack. Both legs are placed between roller pads so that the front pad is against your hip and the rear against the back of your thigh. Grip handhold with an underarm grip and elbows at right angles. Rest head on headrest. Moving from the hips slowly extend both legs as far back as possible. Hold briefly and slowly return legs to starting position without setting down the weights. Repeat until a full movement is no longer possible.

Muscles:

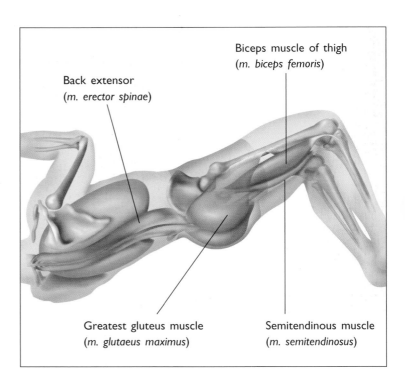

Back extensor
(*m. erector spinae*)

Biceps muscle of thigh
(*m. biceps femoris*)

Greatest gluteus muscle
(*m. glutaeus maximus*)

Semitendinous muscle
(*m. semitendinosus*)

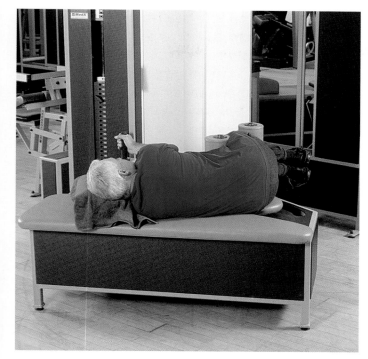

Important:
Do not use momentum to complete movement and extend both legs evenly from hips.

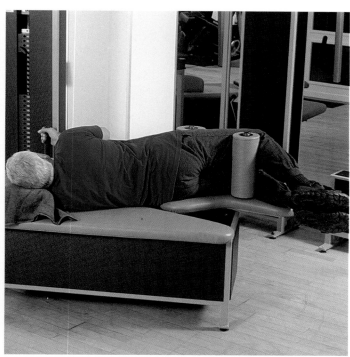

Torso flexion

Select weight. Lie on your side facing the weight stack. Place legs between roller pads so that front pad is above the knee, the upper rear pad under the buttocks and the lower rear pad against your calves. Grip handhold with an overarm grip, stretch your arms and rest head on headrest. Moving from the hip bring knees slowly to your chest. Hold curled-up position briefly and then return knees slowly to starting position without setting down the weights. Repeat until a full movement is no longer possible.

Muscles:

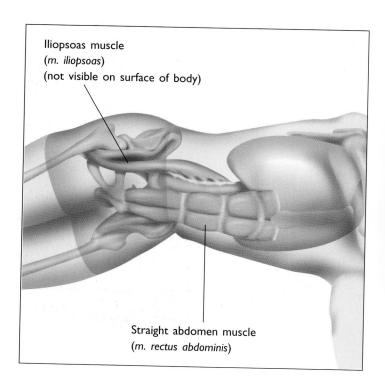

Iliopsoas muscle
(*m. iliopsoas*)
(not visible on surface of body)

Straight abdomen muscle
(*m. rectus abdominis*)

Important:
Hold yourself in position by locking your calves firmly around lower rear pad.

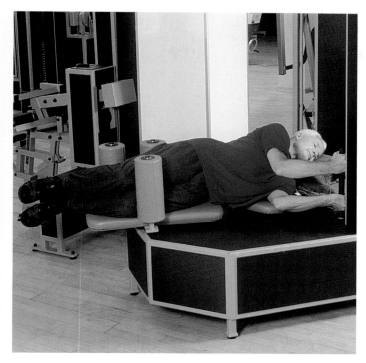

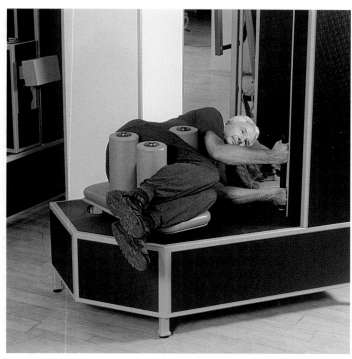

Abductor

Select weight. Adjust backrest. Sit down and adjust thigh pads. Fasten belt. Slowly press thighs against pads and open legs as far as possible. Hold briefly and then slowly return legs to starting position without setting down the weights. Repeat until a full movement is no longer possible. Keep upper body and arms relaxed during entire exercise.

Muscles:

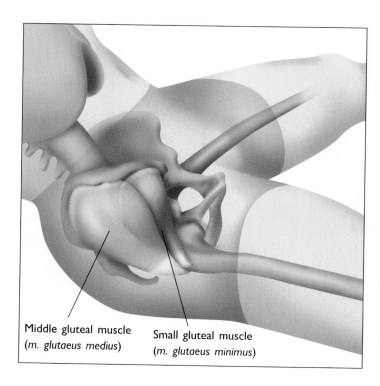

Middle gluteal muscle
(*m. glutaeus medius*)

Small gluteal muscle
(*m. glutaeus minimus*)

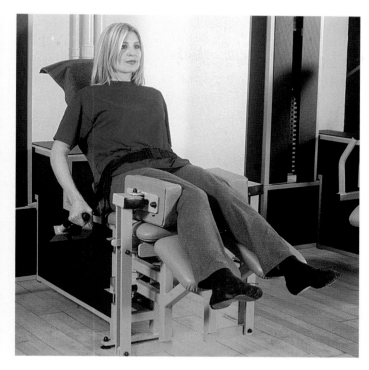

Important:
Do not slide forward
during exercise.

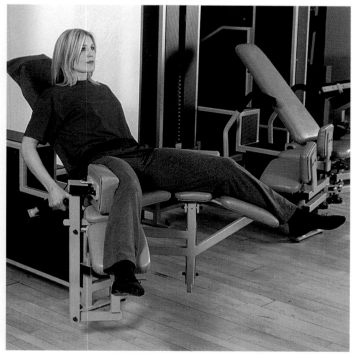

Adductor

Select weight and adjust backrest. Sit down and press down handholds. Place insides of thighs against pads. Slowly let go of handholds and lean back. Using thighs slowly bring knees together, hold this postion briefly and then slowly return to starting position. Repeat until a full movement is no longer possible. To exit machine press down on handholds.

Muscles:

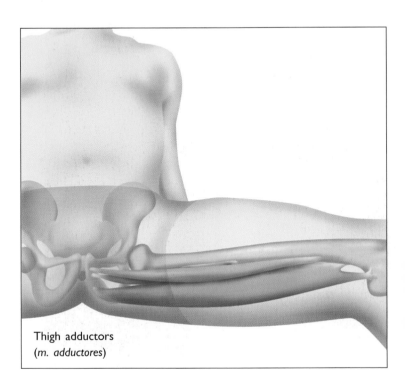

Thigh adductors
(*m. adductores*)

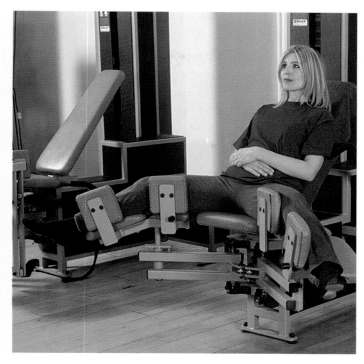

Important:
Do not bow legs
during the exercise.

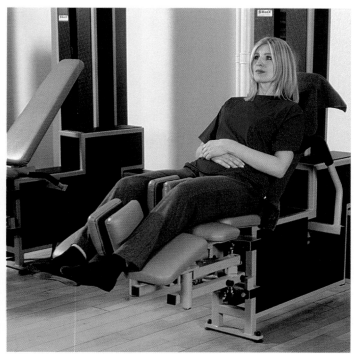

Leg extension

Select weight. Adjust backrest so that knees are in line with pivot of machine. Sit in machine with your lower legs positioned behind lever arm, your knees slightly apart and your feet flexed. Fasten belt and place hands on handholds. Moving from the knees slowly extend both legs until they are fully stretched. Hold briefly. Slowly lower legs to starting position without allowing the weight to touch down. Repeat until a full movement is no longer possible.

Muscles:

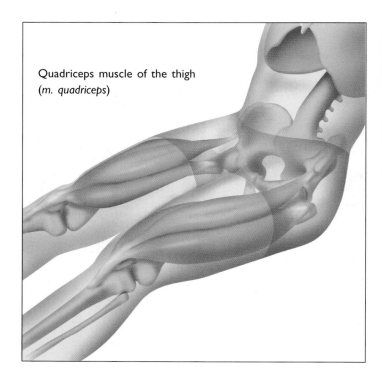

Quadriceps muscle of the thigh
(*m. quadriceps*)

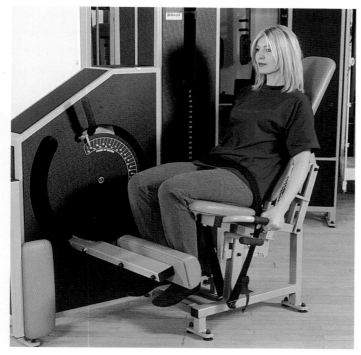

Important:
During entire exercise keep back straight and neck and facial muscles relaxed.

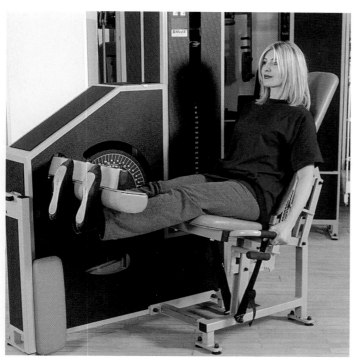

Prone leg curl

Select weight. Lie face down on pad with feet under the pad of the lever arm. Make sure that knees are in line with pivot of machine. Grip both handholds. Bend knees and slowly raise heels towards your buttocks. Hold this position briefly and then slowly lower legs to the starting position without setting down the weights. Repeat until a full movement is no longer possible.

Muscles:

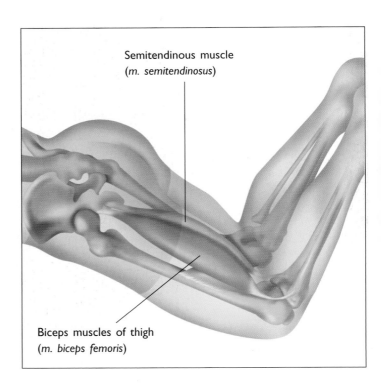

Semitendinous muscle
(*m. semitendinosus*)

Biceps muscles of thigh
(*m. biceps femoris*)

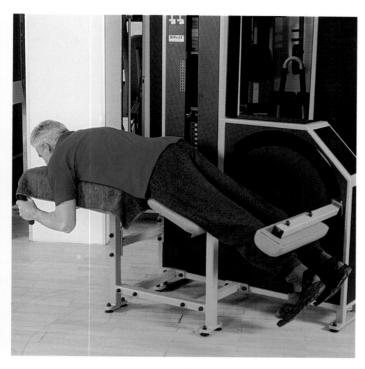

Important:
During the entire exercise feet should be flexed.

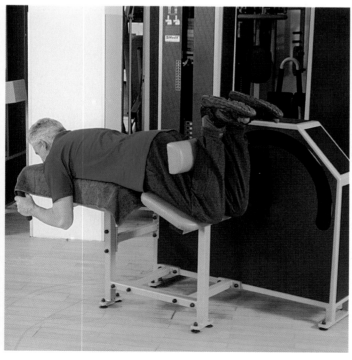

Leg press

Select weight. Adjust seat position, angle of backrest and shoulder pad. Sit in machine. Place both feet on foot plate and grip handholds. Slowly extend both legs, but stop short of locking your knees. Hold briefly and then return to starting position without setting down the weights. Repeat until a full movement is no longer possible.

Muscles:

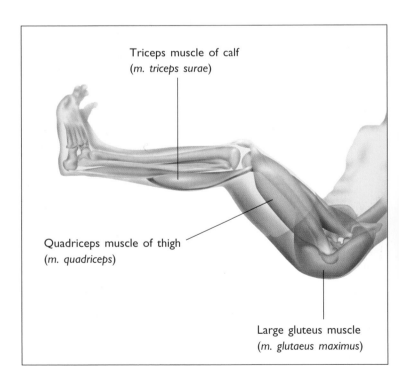

Triceps muscle of calf
(*m. triceps surae*)

Quadriceps muscle of thigh
(*m. quadriceps*)

Large gluteus muscle
(*m. glutaeus maximus*)

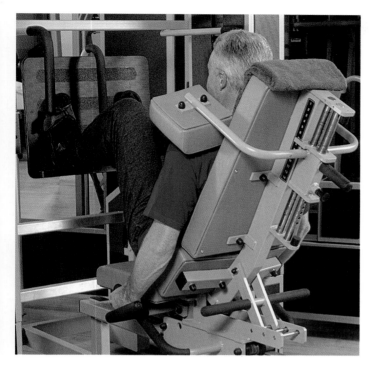

Important:
Knees should be aligned with toes throughout exercise.

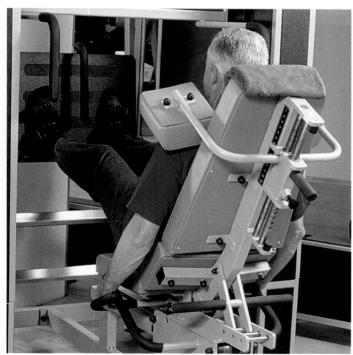

Seated leg curl

Adjust backrest. Remove pins from weight stack. Sit in machine and with right hand push handgrip of lever arm forward and down. Now place both legs between the pads. Stretch legs and with your right hand pull back handgrip of lever arm as far as possible. Select weight. Place hands on side handholds. Bend legs at knee trying to get heels as close to buttocks as possible. Hold briefly and then return legs to starting position without allowing weight to touch down. Repeat until a full movement is no longer possible.

Muscles:

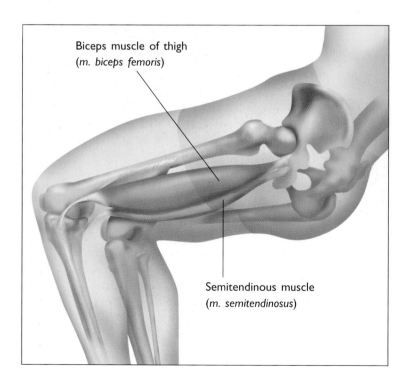

Biceps muscle of thigh
(*m. biceps femoris*)

Semitendinous muscle
(*m. semitendinosus*)

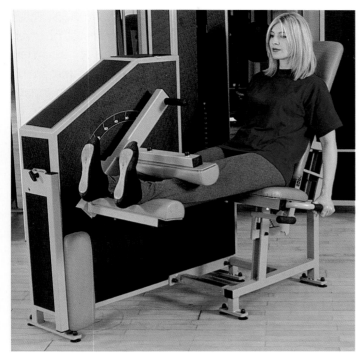

Important:
During entire exercise feet should be flexed and back should not arch.

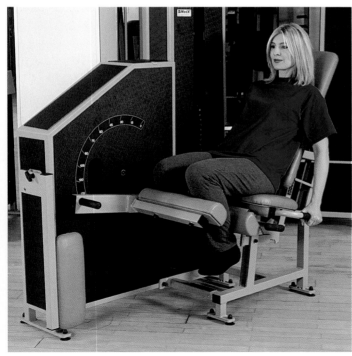

Tibia dorsiflexion

Select weight. Raise knee pad so that foot slides easily under foot pad. Return lower leg to vertical position and knee pad to original position. Raise foot slowly at ankle. Hold the raised position briefly and then slowly lower foot. Repeat until a full movement is no longer possible.

Muscles:

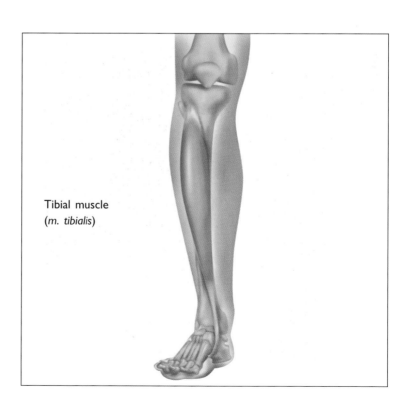

Tibial muscle
(*m. tibialis*)

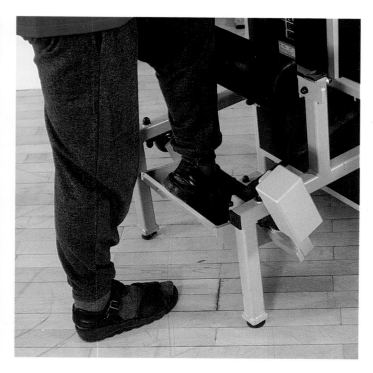

Important:
Lower weight
carefully during
extension phase.

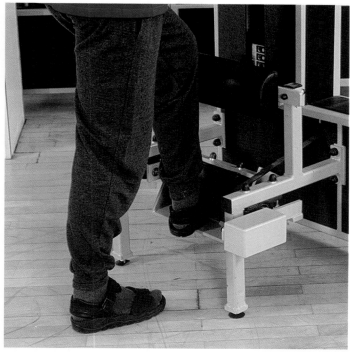

Pullover

Select weight. Adjust seat height so that shoulders are 3cm below pivot of machine. Adjust backrest and elbow pads and fasten belt. Press down on pedals. Place elbows on pads and rest hands on handholds.

Carefully remove feet from pedals so that your upper arms take the full load. Slowly give way to load until your upper arms are behind your head. Now press elbows down in a semi-circle until machine reaches its stop position. Hold briefly. Repeat until a full movement is no longer possible. Do not move head or torso during exercise.

Muscles:

Latissimus dorsi muscle
(*m. latissimus dorsi*)

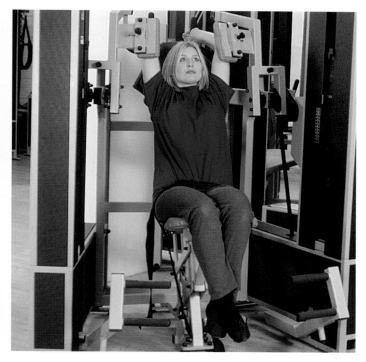

Important:
During entire exercise upper body should remain straight and in contact with backrest. Relax hands and do all the work through your upper arms.

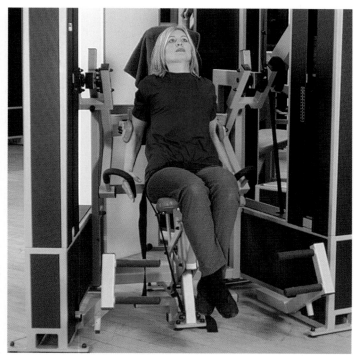

Torso arm

Select weight. Adjust seat. Fasten belt and grip handholds above you. Lean slightly forward. Pull handholds down until hands are level with shoulders making sure that elbows do not move forward. Hold briefly and then slowly return to starting position. Repeat until a full movement is no longer possible. Weights should not touch down when arms are in extended position. If they do, lower seat position.

Muscles:

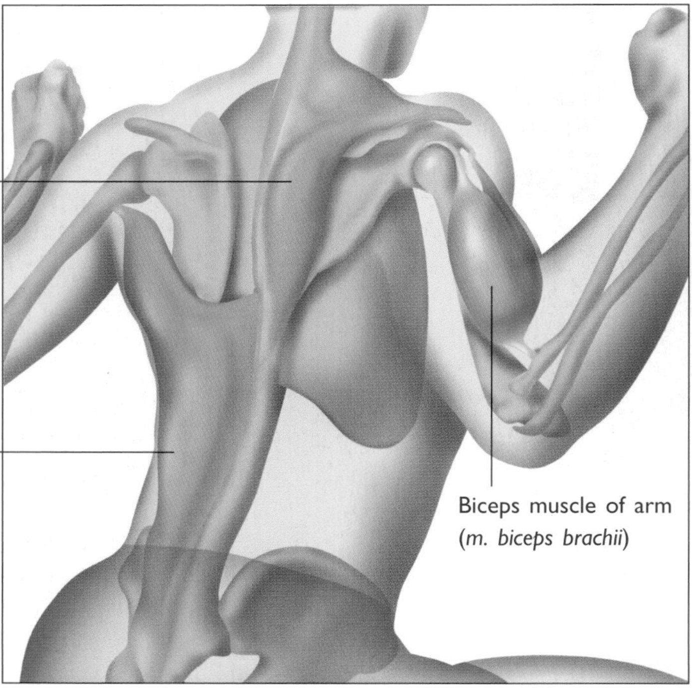

Trapezius muscle
(*m. trapezius*),
lower section

Latissimus dorsi muscle
(*m. latissimus dorsi*)

Biceps muscle of arm
(*m. biceps brachii*)

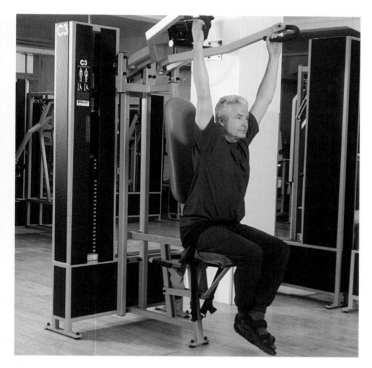

Important:
Keep back straight
and lean forward.

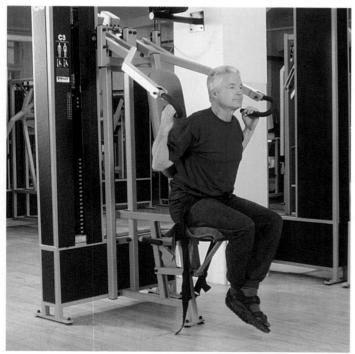

Rowing torso

Select weight. Adjust seat. Sit with back to weight stack. Adjust chest pad, release lever arms, bring them forward and re-engage them. Place elbows in arm pads and keep arms crossed with elbows at right angles. Press arms back as far as possible. Keep arms in one plane parallel with the floor. Hold briefly and then return to starting position without setting down the weights. Repeat until a full movement is no longer possible.

Muscles:

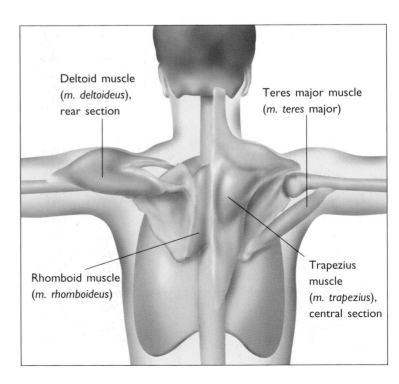

Deltoid muscle
(*m. deltoideus*),
rear section

Teres major muscle
(*m. teres* major)

Rhomboid muscle
(*m. rhomboideus*)

Trapezius
muscle
(*m. trapezius*),
central section

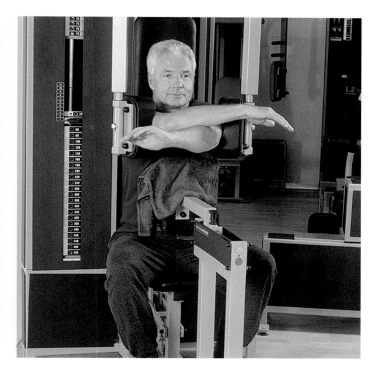

Important:
Keep chest in contact with chest pad.

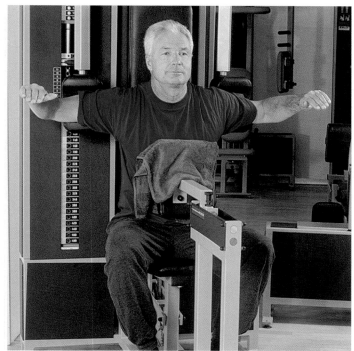

C7 **Row**

Select weight. Adjust seat position so that you can just reach handholds. Pull elbows back as far as possible keeping head and shoulders still. Hold briefly and then return slowly to starting position. Repeat until a full movement is no longer possible.

During entire exercise head should remain relaxed and straight and chest should remain in contact with pad. Do not let weight touch down in the extended position. If it does, adjust chest pad.

Muscles:

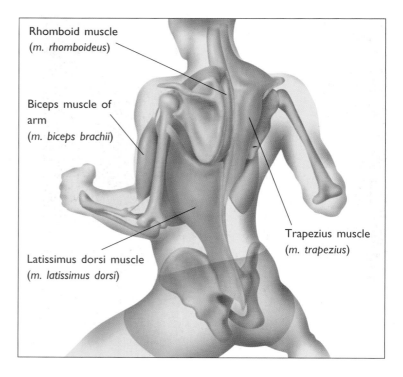

Rhomboid muscle
(*m. rhomboideus*)

Biceps muscle of
arm
(*m. biceps brachii*)

Trapezius muscle
(*m. trapezius*)

Latissimus dorsi muscle
(*m. latissimus dorsi*)

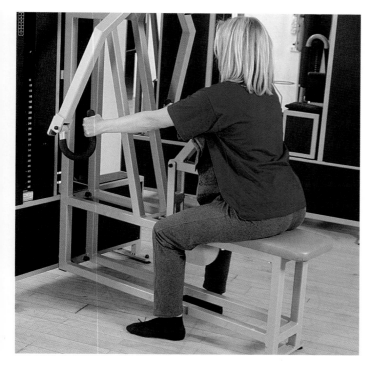

Important:
Keep neck muscles
relaxed and do not
bend wrists.

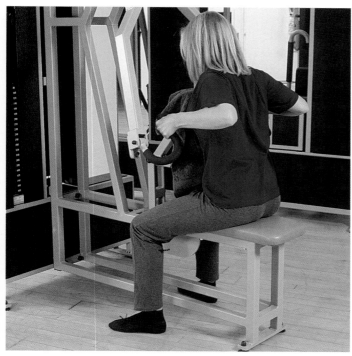

Arm cross

Select weight. Adjust backrest and armpads. Sit down and rest lower arms on arm pad keeping upper arms parallel with floor. Lightly grip handholds or upper edge of arm pads. Using your lower arms press lever arms forward until they touch. Hold this position briefly and then slowly return to starting position. Repeat until a full movement is no longer possible.

Muscles:

Greater pectoral muscle
(*m. pectoralis* major)

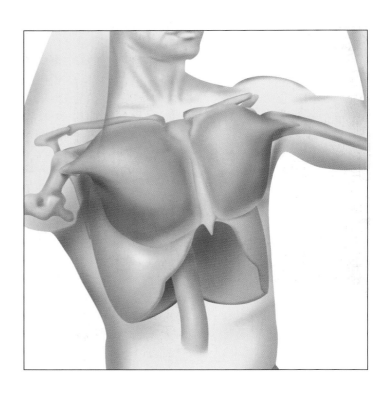

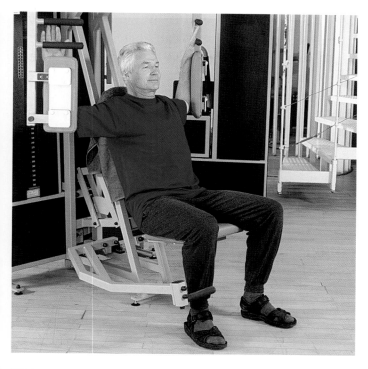

Important:
Do not hollow your back. Keep hands loosely on handholds.

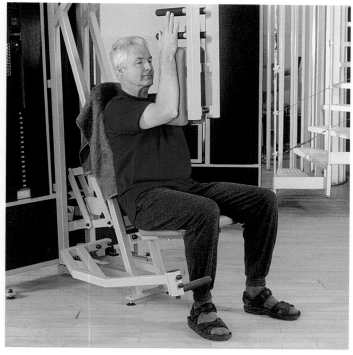

Chest press

Select weight. Adjust seat height and backrest. Press forward extending arms. Hold position briefly and slowly return to starting position without setting down the weights. Repeat until a full movement is no longer possible.

Muscles:

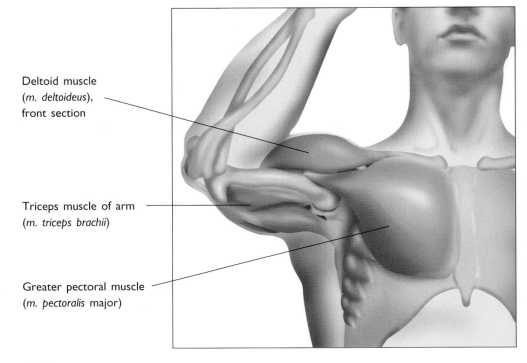

Deltoid muscle
(*m. deltoideus*),
front section

Triceps muscle of arm
(*m. triceps brachii*)

Greater pectoral muscle
(*m. pectoralis* major)

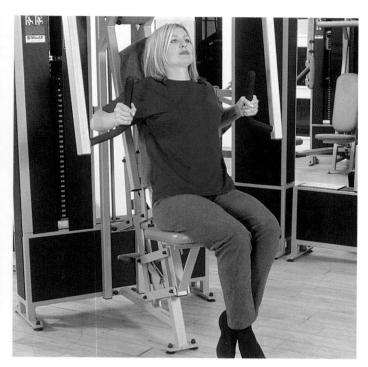

Important:
Do not hollow back
and do not fully
stretch your arms.
Elbows point
outward during
movement.

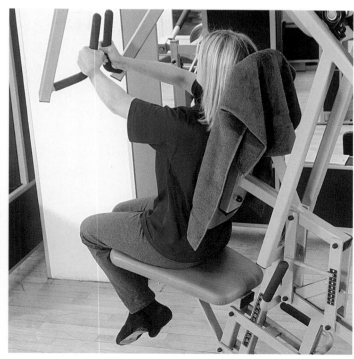

Seated dip

Select weight. Adjust seat and handholds. Fasten belt and grip handholds. Lean slightly forward. Press down on handholds keeping elbows pointing outwards. Do not straighten arms fully but stop with elbows still slightly bent. Slowly return arms to starting position. Repeat until a full movement is no longer possible.

Muscles:

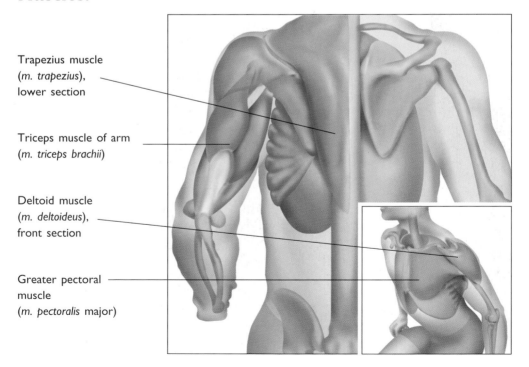

Trapezius muscle (*m. trapezius*), lower section

Triceps muscle of arm (*m. triceps brachii*)

Deltoid muscle (*m. deltoideus*), front section

Greater pectoral muscle (*m. pectoralis* major)

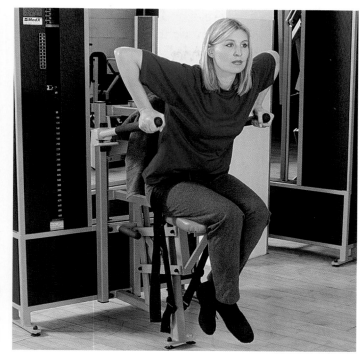

Important:
Make sure that elbows remain in line with body and not behind it.

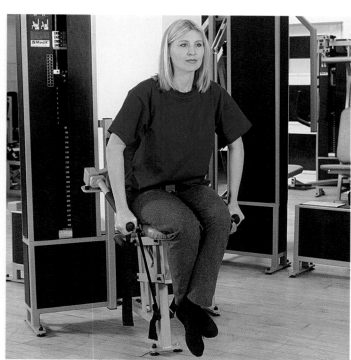

Neck press

Select weight. Adjust seat height and backrest. Push horizontal handholds upwards but do not straighten arms fully locking elbows. Hold position briefly and then slowly return to starting position. Repeat until a full movement is no longer possible.

Muscles:

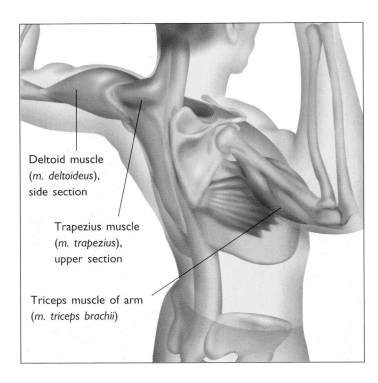

Deltoid muscle
(*m. deltoideus*),
side section

Trapezius muscle
(*m. trapezius*),
upper section

Triceps muscle of arm
(*m. triceps brachii*)

Important:
Keep back straight.

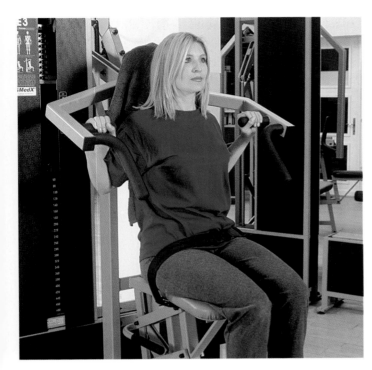

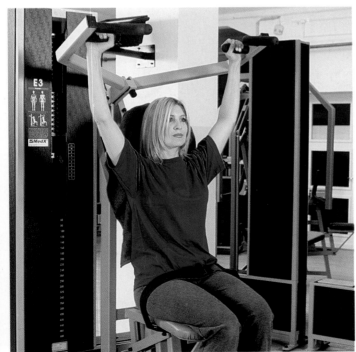

Lateral raise

Select weight. Adjust seat height and backrest. After sitting down, adjust handholds. Grip handholds so that elbows are resting on the pads. Using the elbows press pads sideways and up. Hold position briefly and then slowly return to the starting position without setting down the weights. Repeat until a full movement is no longer possible.

The lever arm angle can be varied. The wider the angle the less the load on the shoulders and the greater the range of motion. At the narrowest angle setting the upper arms should not go beyond the horizontal position.

Muscles:

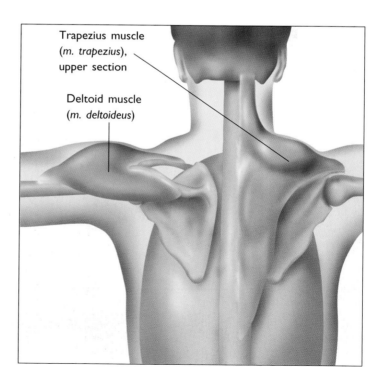

Trapezius muscle
(*m. trapezius*),
upper section

Deltoid muscle
(*m. deltoideus*)

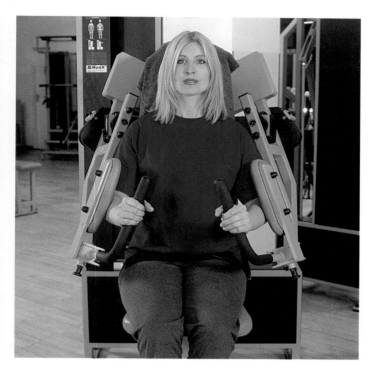

Important:
Do not raise shoulders.

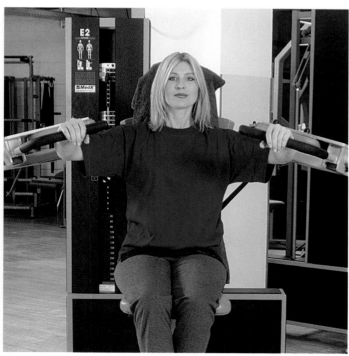

Overhead press

Select weight. Adjust seat and backrest. Sit down and grip forward-pointing handholds. Push upwards but do not straighten arms fully locking elbows. Hold position briefly and then slowly return to starting position. Repeat until a full movement is no longer possible.

Muscles:

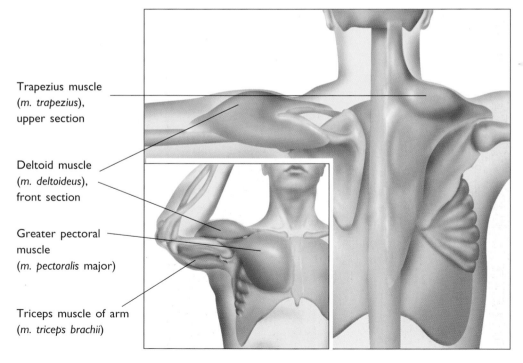

Trapezius muscle
(*m. trapezius*),
upper section

Deltoid muscle
(*m. deltoideus*),
front section

Greater pectoral
muscle
(*m. pectoralis* major)

Triceps muscle of arm
(*m. triceps brachii*)

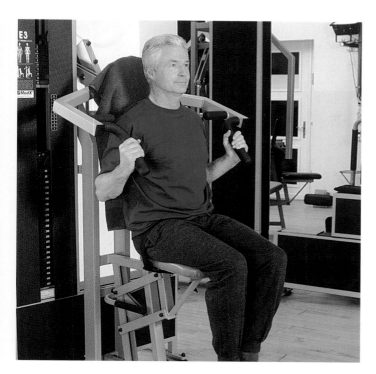

Important:
Keep back straight.

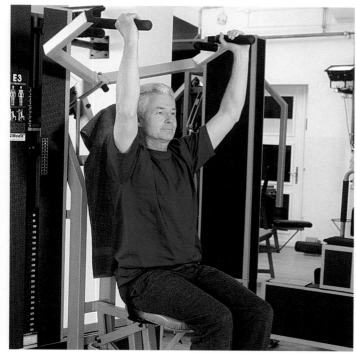

Internal rotation-shoulder

Select weight. Adjust seat height. Rotate lever arm to the back with handhold facing up. Sit down and grip handhold so that your lower arm is at right angles to your upper arm with the back of your hand just behind your ear. Now rotate arm forward and down. Hold briefly in the down position and then return arm to starting position. Repeat until a full movement is no longer possible. Turn seat to opposite direction and repeat exercise for other shoulder.

Muscles:

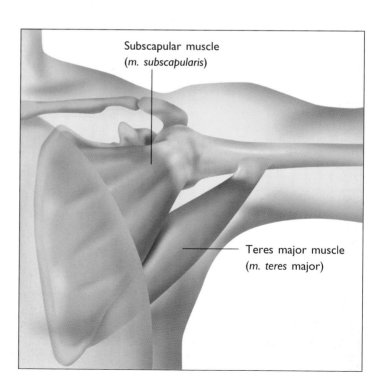

Subscapular muscle
(*m. subscapularis*)

Teres major muscle
(*m. teres* major)

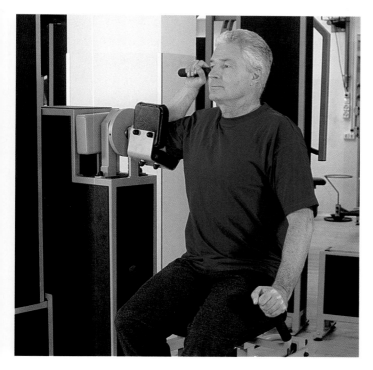

Important:
Do not raise shoulders during exercise and keep both shoulders in contact with the backrest. Keep wrist straight.

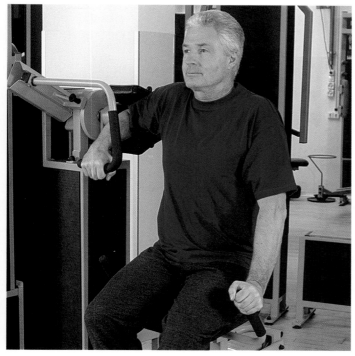

Select weight. Adjust seat height. Rotate lever arm to front with handhold facing down. Grip handhold so that lower arm is at right angles to upper arm. Your hand should be just below chest with back of hand facing upward. Now rotate arm up and back. Hold briefly in the up position and then return arm to starting position. Repeat until a full movement is no longer possible. Turn seat to opposite direction and repeat exercise for other shoulder.

Muscles:

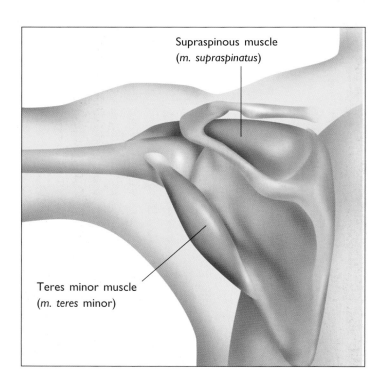

Supraspinous muscle
(*m. supraspinatus*)

Teres minor muscle
(*m. teres minor*)

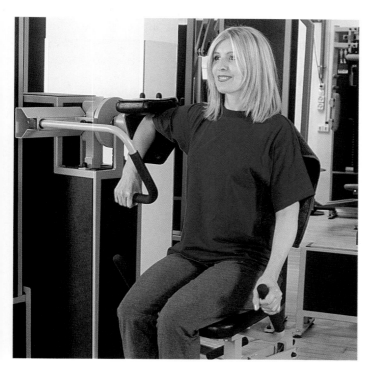

Important:
Do not raise shoulders during exercise and keep both shoulders in contact with the backrest. Keep wrist straight.

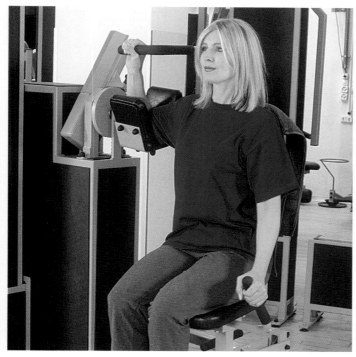

Rotary torso

Sit in machine and select weight. Adjust foot platform. Place feet on foot platform so that your lower legs are positioned squarely on the pads. Now hook your right elbow behind the roller pad and with your left hand raise overhead fixing lever. Rotate your upper body as far to the left as possible and let fixing lever reengage. Then hook your left elbow behind the other roller pad and rotate upper body slowly to the right. Back and pelvis must remain in contact with the pads. Hold end position briefly and return upper body to starting position without setting down the weights. Repeat until a full movement is no longer possible.

To train antagonist muscle rotate upper body back to starting position until weight touches down. Release fixing lever over your head and with lever disengaged rotate upper body in the opposite direction and let the fixing lever re-engage.

Muscles:

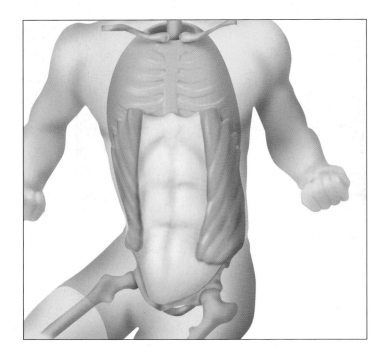

Oblique muscles of the abdomen
(*mm. obliqui abdomini*)

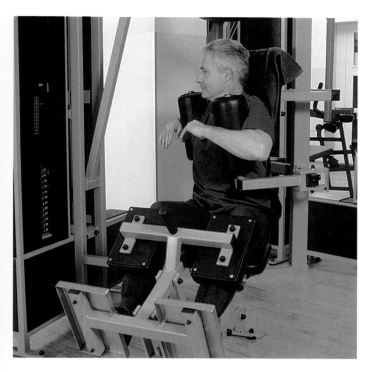

Important:
During entire exercise keep your upper body straight, your feet still and your pelvis in a fixed position.

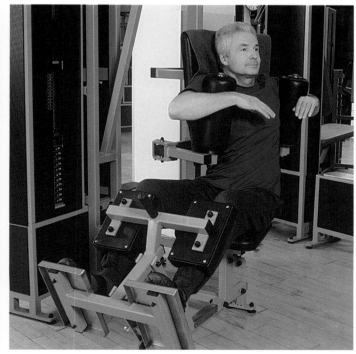

Abdominal

Sit in machine. Select weight. Push your knees apart slightly with the leg-splay mechanism. Grip the roller pad and pull it over your head and down to your chest. Then rest your upper arms on roller pad, keeping your hands by the side of your head. Curl upper body downward in the navel area. Hold the fully contracted position briefly and then straighten up but do not let the weight touch down. Repeat until a full movement is no longer possible.

Muscles:

Straight muscle of abdomen
(*m. rectus abdominis*)

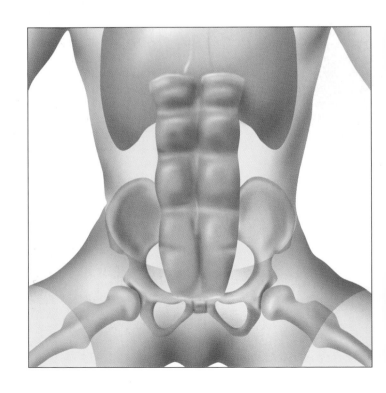

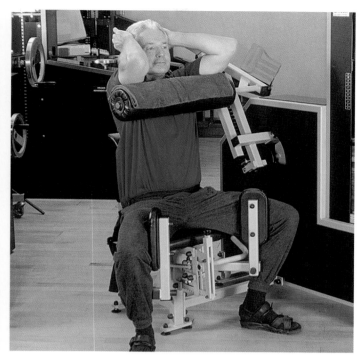

Important:
Make sure your lower back remains in contact with the pad throughout the exercise.

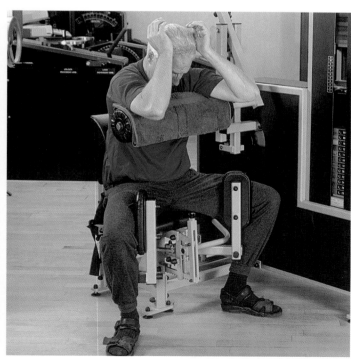

Lower back

Select weight. Adjust foot platform and knee pad. Sit in machine. Grip handholds adjacent to seat and straighten your legs and arms in order to push yourself out of seat. Place feet properly on foot platform and knees behind knee pad. Lower yourself back into the seat. Bend forward and grip the two handholds under the seat. Using your thumb press button on right handhold and raise both handholds. As soon as backrest touches your fully flexed back release button and lever arm engages with backrest. Cross your arms over chest and slowly straighten upper body until back is hollowed. Make sure your buttocks remain in contact with the seat. Hold position briefly and then slowly return upper body to its starting position without setting down the weights. Repeat until a full movement is no longer possible.

End exercise from the forward position: grip both handholds and press button to release lever arm of backrest.

Muscles:

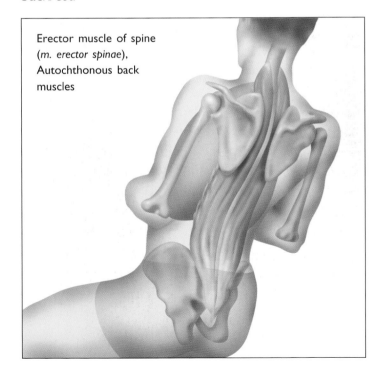

Erector muscle of spine
(*m. erector spinae*),
Autochthonous back
muscles

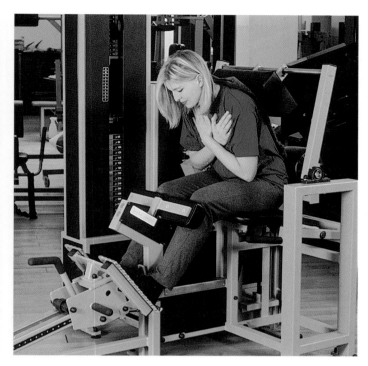

Important:
Make sure that your
buttocks remain on
seat.

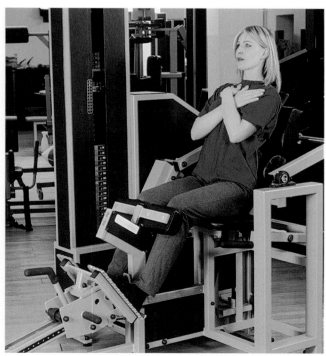

Neck & shoulder

Select weight. Adjust seat position. Sit in machine and place forearms between pads with palms facing upwards and back slightly bent. Press back of hands lightly against lower pad in order to keep forearms steady and straighten back. Slowly raise shoulders as far as possible. Hold briefly and then slowly lower shoulders to starting position without setting down the weights. Repeat until a full movement is no longer possible.

Muscles:

Trapezius muscle
(*m. trapezius*),
upper section

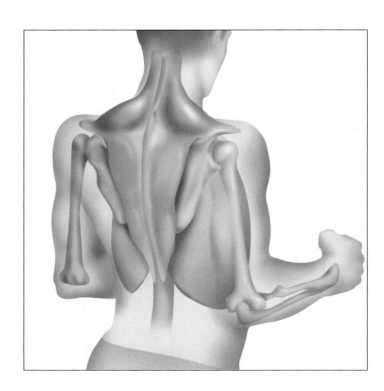

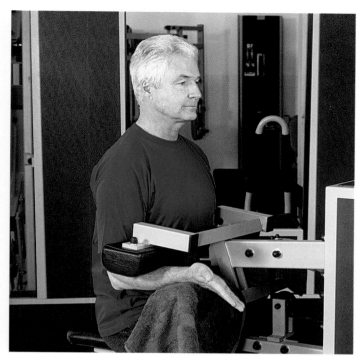

Important:
During the exercise all muscles except the upper section of the trapezius should remain relaxed.

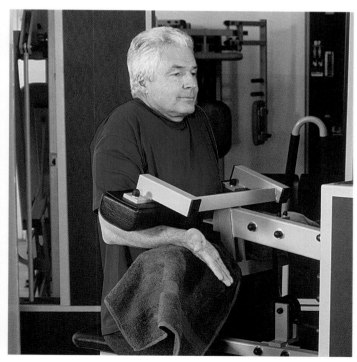

4-way neck—side

Select weight. Adjust seat height, upper body pad and head pad. Sit down facing machine. Grip handholds to steady your position. Using your head push pad towards left shoulder. Keep shoulders relaxed during entire exercise. Hold end position briefly and then slowly return head to starting position without setting down the weights. Repeat until you are unable to do a complete repetition. Then change seat position and exercise other side.

Muscles:

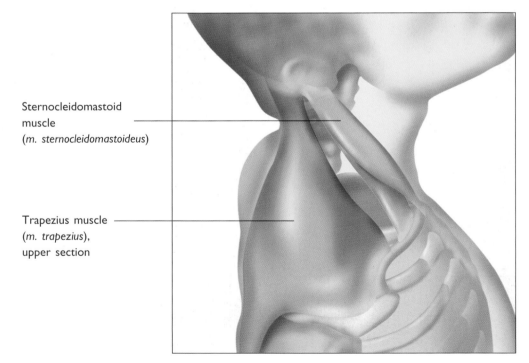

Sternocleidomastoid muscle
(*m. sternocleidomastoideus*)

Trapezius muscle
(*m. trapezius*),
upper section

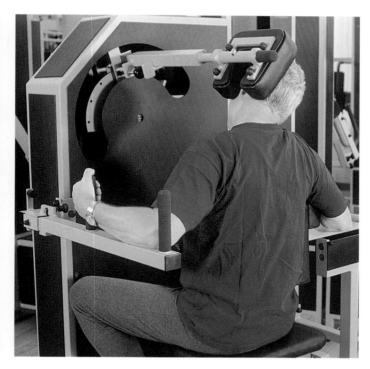

Important:
During entire exercise keep shoulders relaxed and do not swing upper body to and fro.

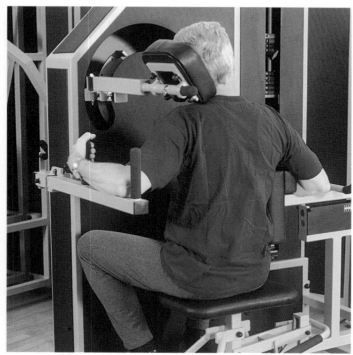

4-way neck—front

Select weight. Adjust seat height, upper body pad and head pad. Sit in machine facing the head pad. Grasp handholds lightly. Using your head press pad forward carefully and slowly. Hold end position briefly and then slowly return head to starting position without setting down the weights. Repeat until a full movement is no longer possible.

Muscles:

Sternocleidomastoid
muscle
(*m. sternocleidomastoideus*)

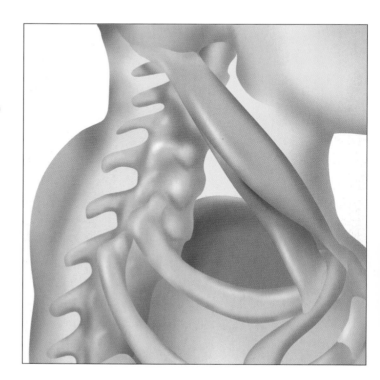

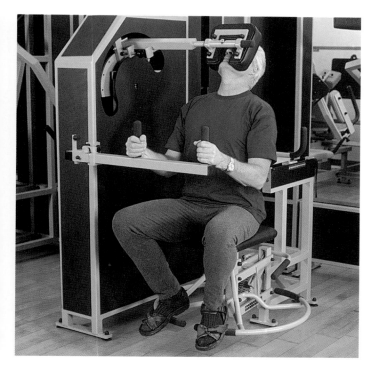

Important:
Lower weight carefully during extension phase. Keep back straight and shoulders relaxed throughout exercise.

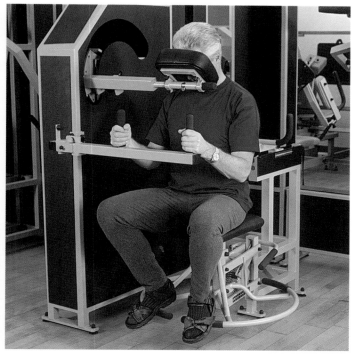

4-way neck—rear

Select weight. Adjust seat height, upper body pad and head pad. Sit in machine so that back of head points to head pad. Grasp handholds. Bend shoulders slightly forward as you bend head back. Do not stretch more than is comfortable. Return to starting position without setting down the weights. Repeat until you are unable to complete a full movement.

Muscles:

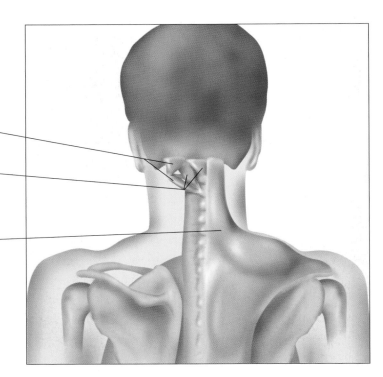

Oblique muscle of head
(*m. obliquus capitis*)

Posterior straight
muscle of head
(*m. rectus capitis*)

Trapezius muscle
(*m. trapezius*),
upper section

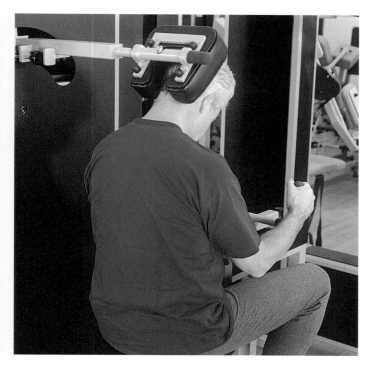

Important:
Work with neck
muscles and not
back muscles.

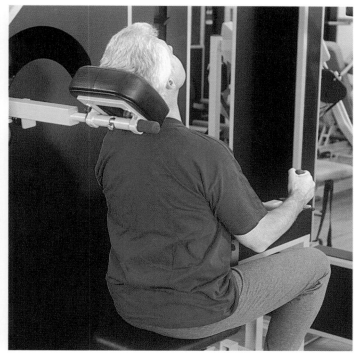

Biceps

Select weight. Adjust seat. Place your elbows between the two pads. Place feet squarely on the floor and not under the seat.

Bend arms as far as possible. Hold position briefly and then return slowly to starting position without setting down the weights. Repeat until a full movement is no longer possible.

Muscles:

Biceps muscle of arm
(*m. biceps brachii*)

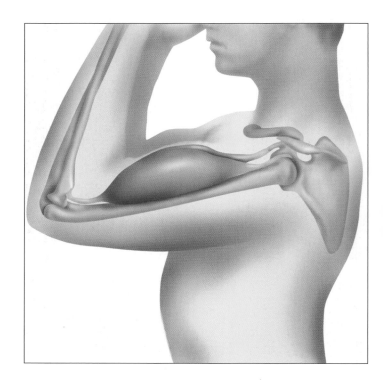

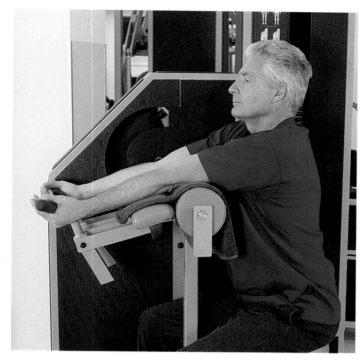

Important:
During entire exercise both upper and lower arms must remain in contact with pads and wrists remain straight. Keep your back straight and your shoulders down.

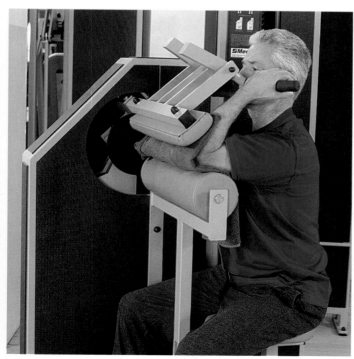

Triceps

Select weight. Adjust seat and arm pad. Use the shoulder pad to secure shoulders as firmly as possible. Straighten arms backward until you reach the stop position. Hold briefly. Slowly return to the starting position but do not allow the weights to touch down. Repeat until a full movement is no longer possible.

Muscles:

Triceps muscle of arm
(*m. triceps brachii*)

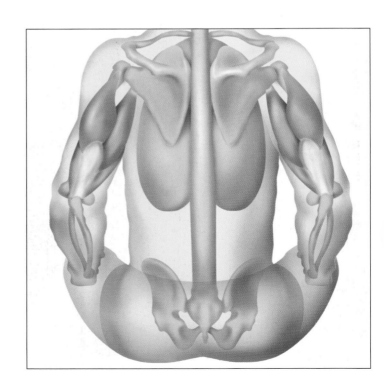

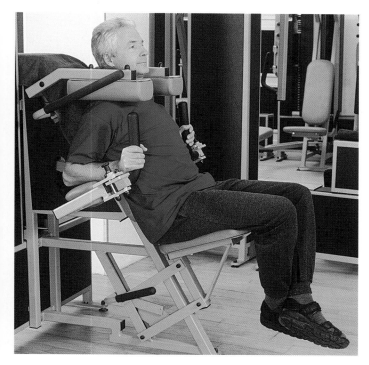

Important:
During the entire exercise lower arms must remain in contact with the pads.

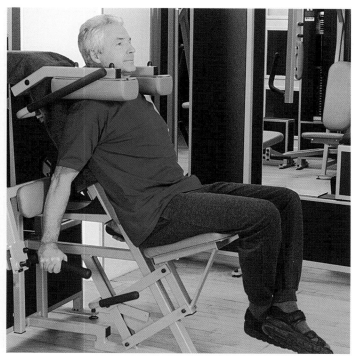

Wrist pronation

Select weight and adjust seat. Rotate handholds to middle of machine until a resistance is met. Now grip handholds with back of hands facing down. Rotate both handholds inward as far as possible. Hold position briefly and then return hands to starting position without setting down the weights. Repeat until a full movement is no longer possible.

Muscles:

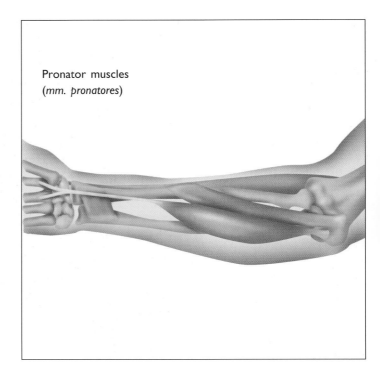

Pronator muscles
(*mm. pronatores*)

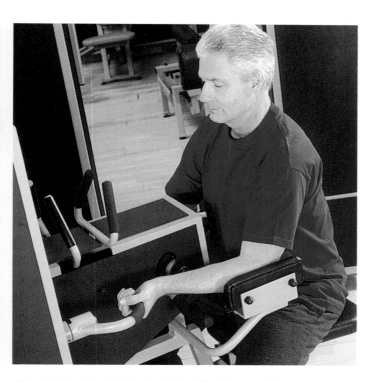

Important:
Lower arms must remain on the pads.

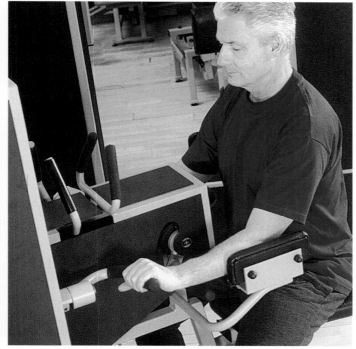

Wrist supination

Select weight and adjust seat. Rotate handholds outward until a resistance is met. Grip handholds with back of hands facing up. Now rotate both handholds outward as far as possible. Hold position briefly and then return to starting position without setting down the weights. Repeat until a full movement is no longer possible.

Muscles:

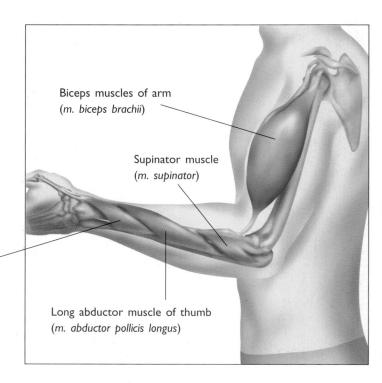

Biceps muscles of arm
(*m. biceps brachii*)

Supinator muscle
(*m. supinator*)

Short extensor muscle of thumb
(*m. extensor pollicis brevis*)

Long abductor muscle of thumb
(*m. abductor pollicis longus*)

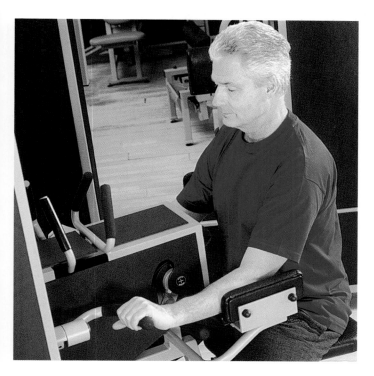

Important:
Lower arms must remain on pads.

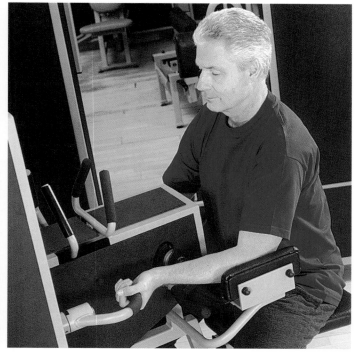

Wrist curl

Select weight and adjust seat. Grip lever arm with back of hand facing down. Make sure that wrists are in line with pivot of lever arm. Lean slightly forward and bend hands up at wrist. Hold highest position briefly and then return hands to starting position without setting down the weights. Repeat until a full movement is no longer possible.

Muscles:

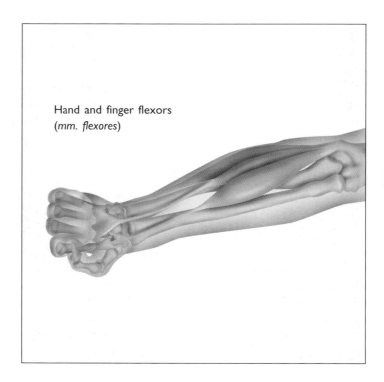

Hand and finger flexors
(*mm. flexores*)

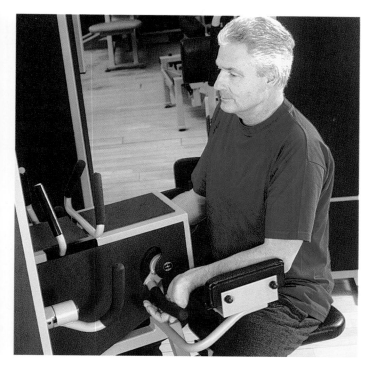

Important:
Keep biceps relaxed
and forearm on pad.

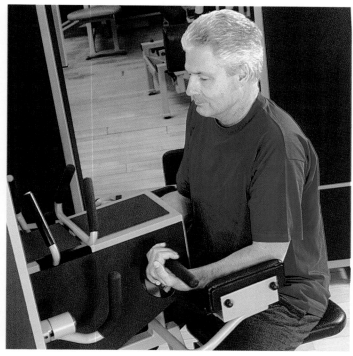

Reverse wrist curl

Select weight and adjust seat. Grip lever arm with back of hand facing up. Using wrists rotate hands towards body. Hold end position briefly and then return hands to starting position without setting down the weights. Repeat until a full movement is no longer possible.

Muscles:

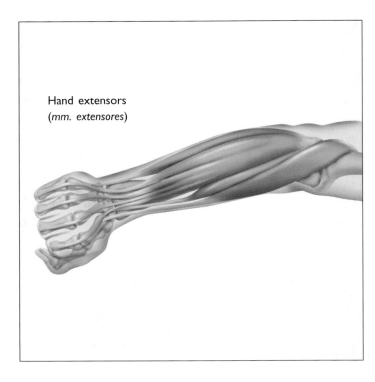

Hand extensors
(*mm. extensores*)

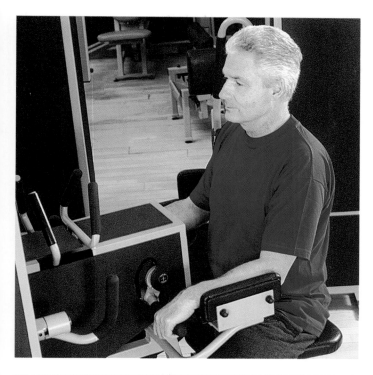

Important:
Keep lower arms on pads.

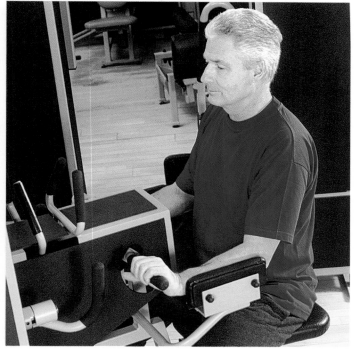

Hand grip

Select weight. Pull the far handholds on top of machine back until your thumbs can grasp the handholds nearer to you. Squeeze both sets of handholds together. Hold position briefly and then slowly return to starting position. Repeat until a full movement is no longer possible.

Muscles:

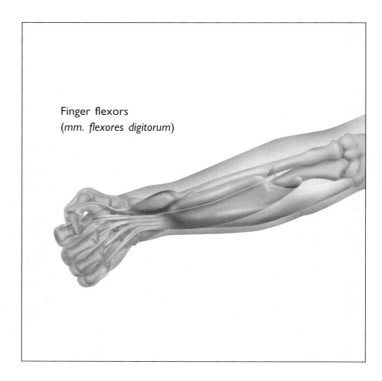

Finger flexors
(*mm. flexores digitorum*)

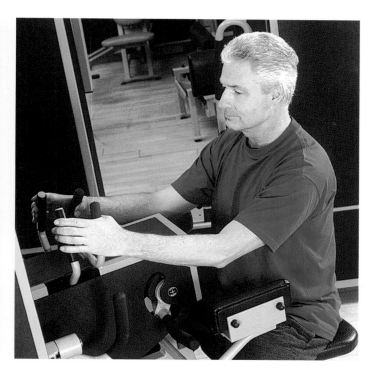

Important:
Make sure your hands are dry.

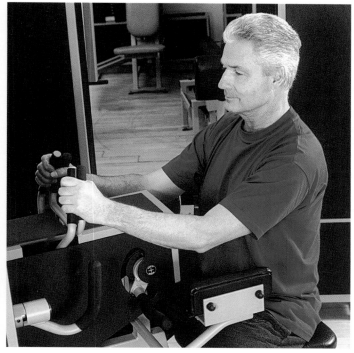

Calf raise

Stand on bottom step on ball of feet. Grip front bar to maintain balance. Raise heels until you are on tiptoes. Hold briefly and then slowly lower heels until fully extended. Repeat until a full movement is no longer possible. The exercise can also be done on one leg. This doubles the load on the calf muscle. The exercise can be further intensified by attaching the belt to the lever arm and selecting an appropriate weight. Repeat.

Muscles:

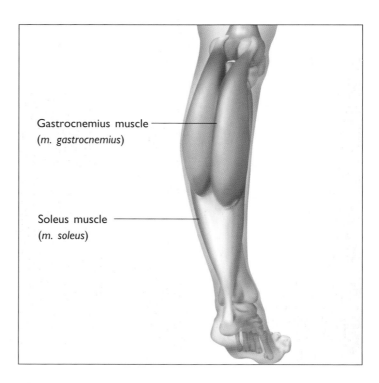

Gastrocnemius muscle
(*m. gastrocnemius*)

Soleus muscle
(*m. soleus*)

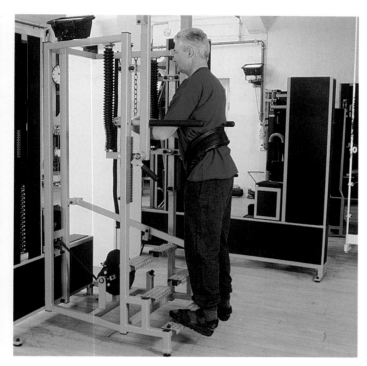

Important:
Make sure that you extend your calves fully and keep body upright.

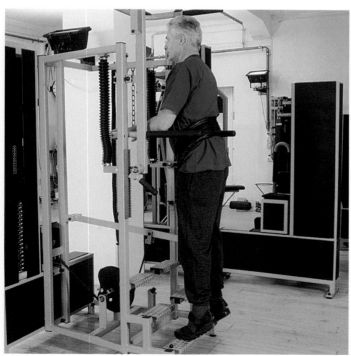

Front chin

Stand on top step and adjust tower unit so that your chin is just above the bar. Grip bar with back of hands facing machine. Slowly lower body until arms are fully extended. Slowly pull yourself back up to starting position. Hold position briefly and repeat until a full movement is no longer possible.

Negative version: just do the first part of the exercise, i.e., lower body into extended position. This movement should take about 10 seconds. Then climb back up to top step and repeat movement.

The exercise can be further intensified by using the belt provided and attaching it to the lever arm and selecting an appropriate weight. Repeat.

Muscles:

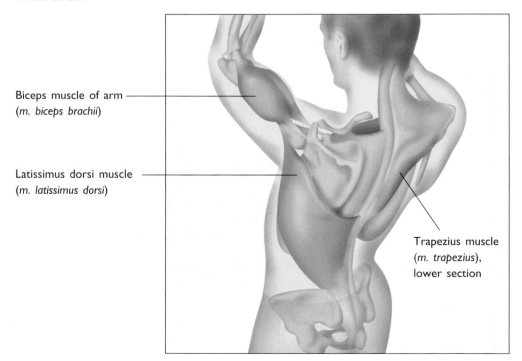

Biceps muscle of arm
(*m. biceps brachii*)

Latissimus dorsi muscle
(*m. latissimus dorsi*)

Trapezius muscle
(*m. trapezius*),
lower section

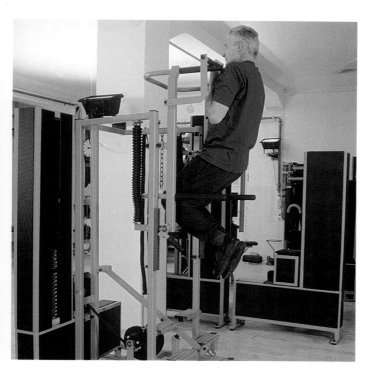

Important:
Do not swing body
or thrash about. Hip
remains straight.

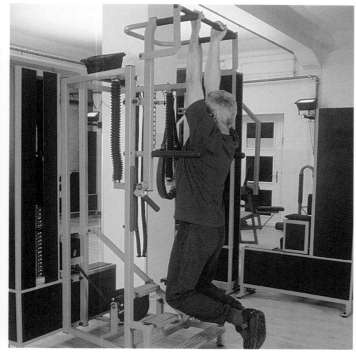

Parallel chin

Fold back cross bar. Stand on top step and adjust tower unit so that your chin is just above the side bars. Grip side bars with back of hands facing outwards. Slowly lower body (about 4 seconds). Pull yourself back up to starting position. Hold position briefly and repeat until a full movement is no longer possible.

Negative version: Just do first part of exercise, i.e. lower body into extended position. This movement should take about 10 seconds. Then climb back up to top step and repeat.

The exercise can be further intensified by using the belt provided and attaching it to the lever arm and selecting an appropriate weight. Repeat.

Muscles:

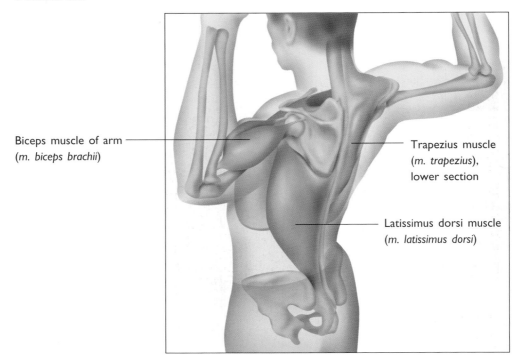

Biceps muscle of arm (*m. biceps brachii*)

Trapezius muscle (*m. trapezius*), lower section

Latissimus dorsi muscle (*m. latissimus dorsi*)

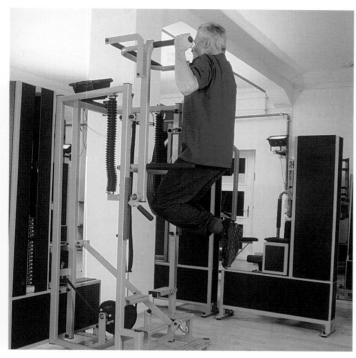

Important:
Make sure that elbows do not move forward during exercise. Hip remains straight.

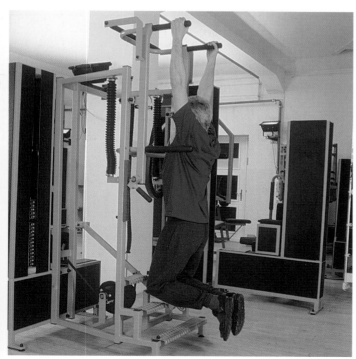

Stand on top step. Grip parallel bars and straighten arms fully and bend lower legs. Bend elbows in order to lower body slowly into fully extended position. Raise body back to starting position without using your feet as support. Do not straighten arms fully and lock elbows. Hold briefly. Repeat until a full movement is no longer possible.

Negative variation: Just do first part of exercise, i.e., lower body into extended position. This movement should take about 10 seconds. Then climb back up to top step and repeat.

The exercise can be further intensified by using the belt provided and attaching it to the lever arm and selecting an appropriate weight. Repeat.

Muscles:

Trapezius muscle
(*m. trapezius*),
lower section

Triceps muscle of arm
(*m. triceps brachii*)

Deltoid muscle
(*m. deltoideus*)
front section

Greater pectoral
muscle
(*m. pectoralis* major)

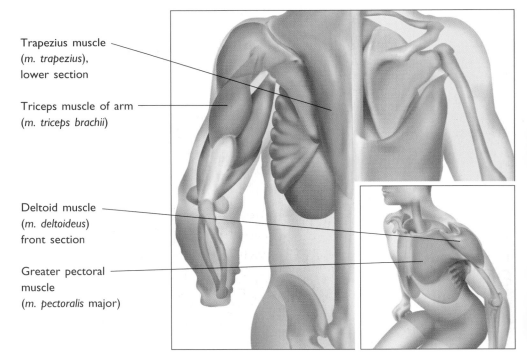

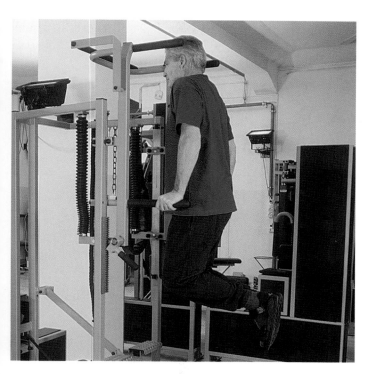

Important:
Make sure that elbows remain in line with body and not behind it.

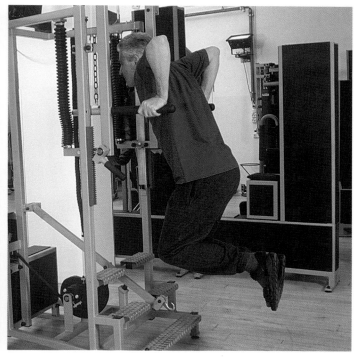

Triceps extension

Select weight. Fix rope to lever arm (or thread towel through weight belt fixed to lever arm). Standing with back to machine hold one end of the rope with one hand and the other with the other hand. Lean slightly forward in order to raise weight slightly from stack. Extend but do not fully straighten arms - make sure movement is smooth. Hold extended position briefly and then slowly lower weight. Repeat until a full movement is no longer possible.

Muscles:

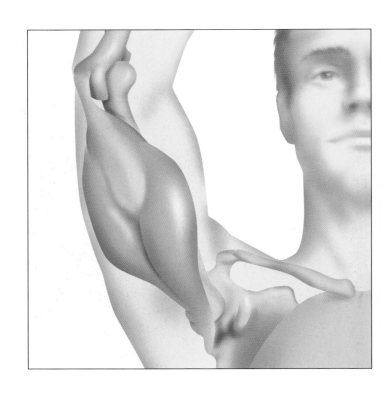

Triceps muscle of arm
(*m. triceps brachii*)

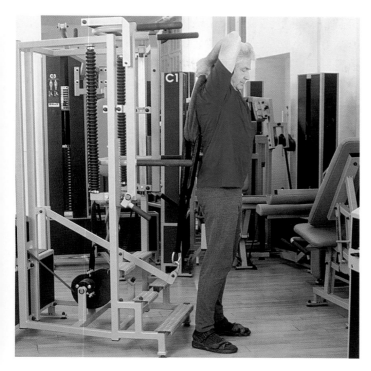

Important:
Make sure you are
standing firmly.

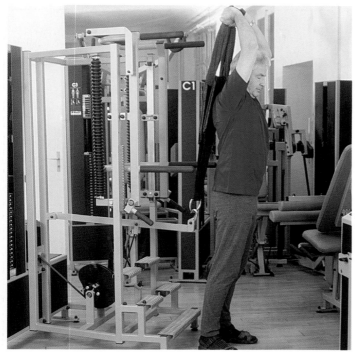

Side bend

Select weight. Attach handhold to lever arm. Grip handhold on lever arm of machine. Stand with one side of body next to machine and grip handhold with one hand. Straighten up, lifting weight. Place other hand on your head. Bend away from machine and then slowly return to starting position. Repeat until a full movement is no longer possible.

Muscles:

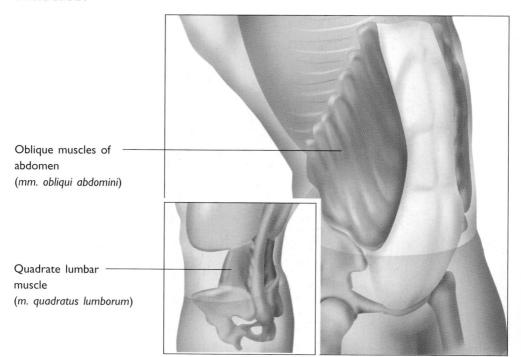

Oblique muscles of
abdomen
(*mm. obliqui abdomini*)

Quadrate lumbar
muscle
(*m. quadratus lumborum*)

BUSINESS REPLY MAIL
FIRST-CLASS MAIL PERMIT NO. 493 BOULDER, CO

POSTAGE WILL BE PAID BY ADDRESSEE

sounds true

PO BOX 8010
BOULDER CO 80306-9886

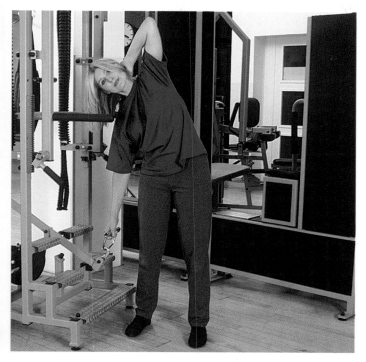

Important:
Bend sideways and not forwards or backwards. Do not swing to and fro. The pivot point should be above the hips. Shoulders remain relaxed.

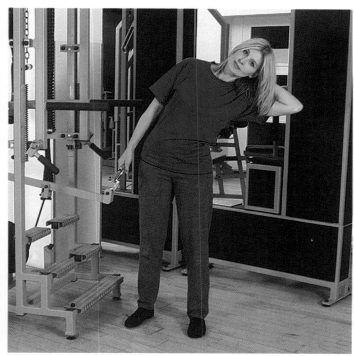

Programmes and methods

Strength-training programmes should be prepared by an instructor with the necessary specialist training. They must reflect individual requirements and objectives. As the following examples of core programmes show, objectives can differ significantly.

Correction programmes

Correction programmes can contain 8–10 exercises

Exercises in a correction programme are particularly important when you first start training. These exercises eliminate intra-muscular imbalances. The number of exercises in a correction programme can range from 8–10 but must include the following five exercises: These exercises are known as the five "correctors" as

1. Hip extension

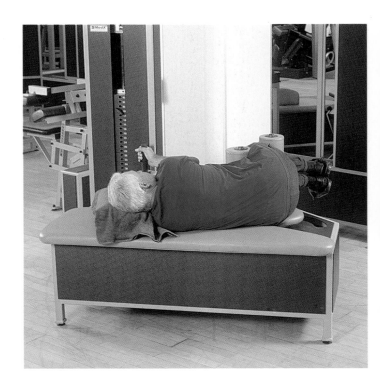

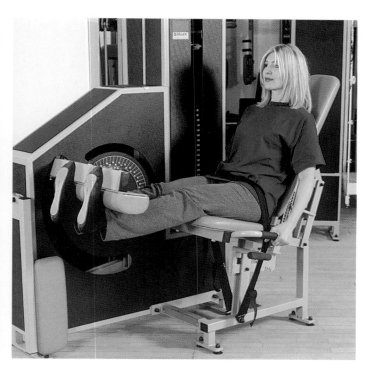

2. Leg extension

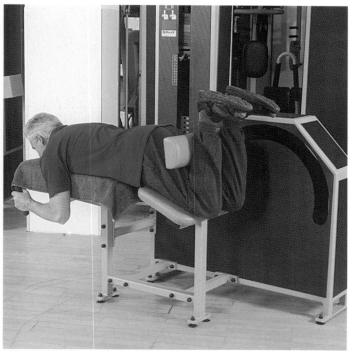

3. Leg curl

157

4. Rotary torso

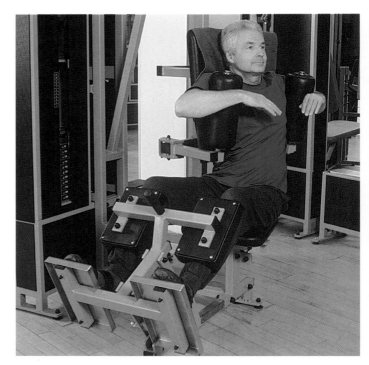

5. Pullover

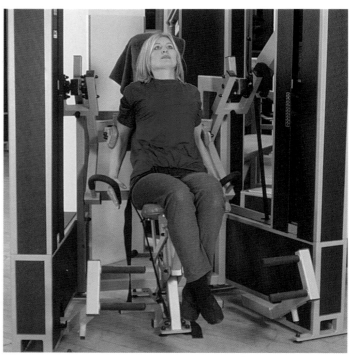

they eliminate distortions in the strength curves of your main muscles. They also increase the mobility of hips, knees, lumbar spine and shoulders. Use them also for the first 3–5 sessions after a longish gap in training. After that you may resume your normal training programme.

The five correctors eliminate intra-muscular imbalances

Maintenance programmes

After a period of regular training—normally 18–24 months—you reach your genetic potential. From then on it is merely a question of maintaining strength with minimum effort. Maintenance programmes are designed to exercise the complete musculoskeletal system in as few exercises as possible. Like correction programmes, maintenance programmes may have up to 10 exercises but must include the following five exercises:

Having achieved your genetic potential you need to maintain that strength

1. Leg press

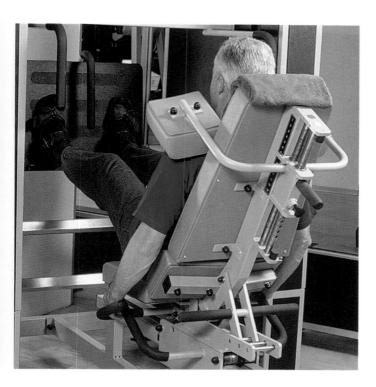

159

2. Overhead press

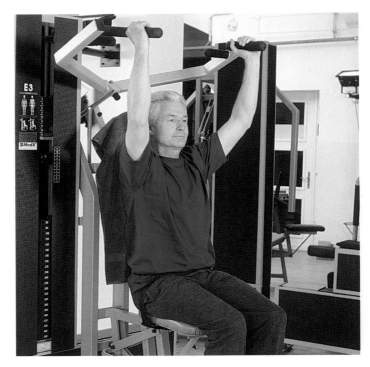

3. Torso arm

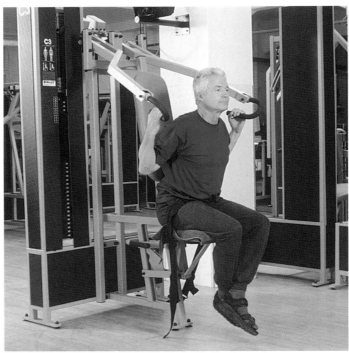

4. Dip

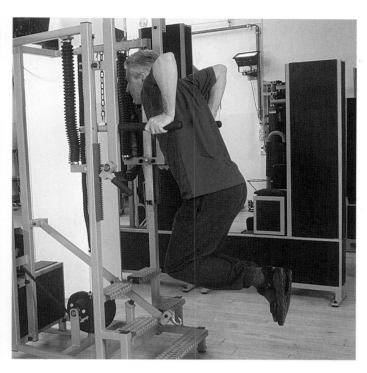

5. Rotary torso

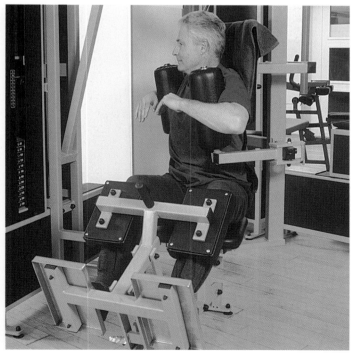

Programme variations

It is not the
programme that
produces the results
but the final seconds
of each exercise

Instructors are frequently asked, "What's the best training programme?" or "May I have a new programme, the old one is no longer working". Many believe that they will only progress with a new programme.

This is an all too human response, an example of evasive action, rather like looking for a key where there is light instead of where it was lost. It is not the programme that produces the results but the individual exercise or rather the last few seconds of an exercise.

The order in which
you do the exercises
is important

There are innumerable examples of "good" training programmes. A programme merely ensures that exercises are done in an appropriate order and provide a balanced routine, so that no muscle is overtaxed or neglected. That is all. Instead of changing your programme it may be more productive to change the method of load.

Pre-fatigue method

With this method you intensify the level of training by doing two exercises without any gap in between. Below are four examples of pre-fatigue programmes:

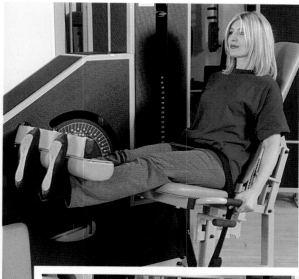

I. Leg extension immediately followed by...

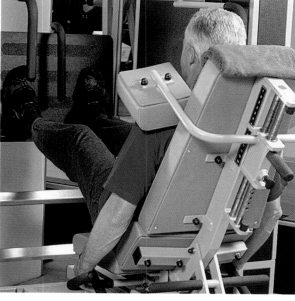

... leg press

The pre-fatigue method only works if you do the two exercises without a gap in-between

Muscles work in a chain containing muscles of different strengths. For example, when you do "chins" your biceps get tired first because they are the weakest muscle in the chain. The strongest muscle in this chain is the *latissimus dorsi* muscle and so "chins" are unable

2. Pullover, immediately followed by...

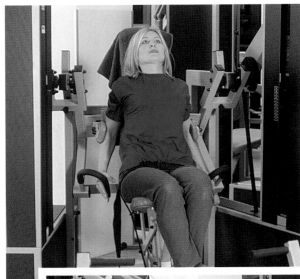

... torso arm

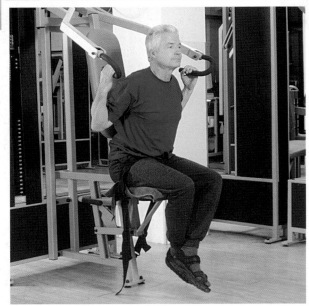

to reach it. In order to increase the efficacy of "chins" you first fatigue the *latissimus dorsi* by doing a pullover. However, this method will only work if both exercises are done without an intervening gap. The same principle can be applied to other muscle groups.

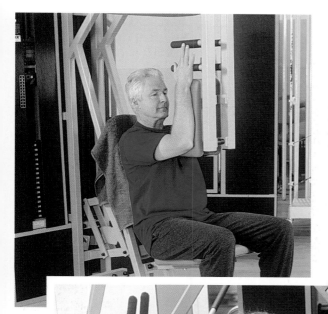

3. Arm cross, immediately followed by...

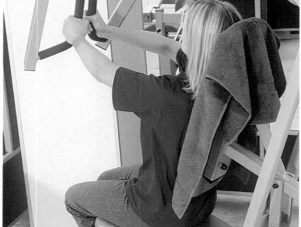

... chest press

This method of training is extremely strenuous and can easily result in overtraining. Rather than using this method for a complete programme it is better to include one or two combination exercises in a "normal" programme.

4. Lateral raise, immediately followed by

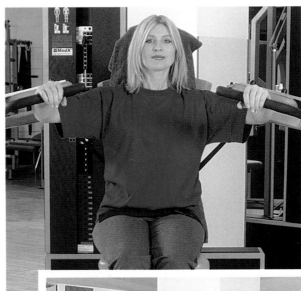

... neck press

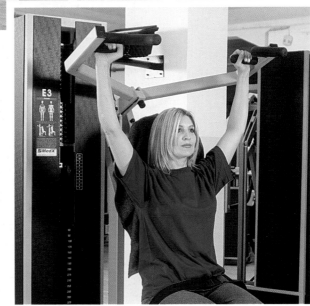

Negative method

"Negative" is the term used to describe the movement to lower a weight and "positive" the movement that lifts it. A negative movement only requires 16% of the energy required for a positive movement. From various studies it would appear that this method is particularly effective. Machine-based training provides good opportunities to exploit this finding as it allows you to select exercises that are "purely negative" or "semi-negative".

Both chins and dips can be done as purely negative exercises: the upper body does no positive work because you use the steps to return to your starting position. The exercise consists solely of lowering the body very slowly (about 10 seconds).

The semi-negative version can be done on all machines without separate lever arms, for example, the leg extension exercise: select a weight about 75% of what you would normally use for this machine (with both legs). Start exercise as usual by straightening both legs at the knees over 4 seconds. Then hold for 1 second before transfering the entire weight to your left leg by lowering your right leg very slightly. The negative movement, i.e., lowering the weight, is done by the left leg over 10 seconds. Alternate the leg you lower under load throughout the exercise.

The energy required for a negative movement is much less than that required for normal exercises. In addition the period under tension is longer and extension more complete

Super-slow method

This method was developed in the early 1980s by a former employee of Nautilus, Ken Hutchins. The difference between super-slow and normal training is one of speed: instead of 4–2–4 seconds each exercise is done to a rhythm of 10–1–4 seconds: the positive phase is extended but the negative phase remains at 4 seconds. When you first start using this method it may help to ask someone to count for you. Alternatively you can time yourself using the clock.

One exercise consists of 4–6 repetitions and so takes 60–90 seconds. Another difference compared with normal training is that each programme has fewer exercises: 5–8 at 100% effort.

When switching from the normal 4–2–4 rhythm to the super-slow method select a weight 10–20% less than your normal weight.

Lift the weight slowly and allow about 10 seconds to contract the muscle fully. Aim to do the positive movement in no less than 8 and no more than 12 seconds. Consciously hold the contracted position for 1 second and then take 4 seconds to return to a point where you can feel the weight is just touching the weight stack. Repeat the exercise. When you are unable to lift the weight with a clean movement, the muscle has had enough! Particular care must be taken whenever the weight is increased. Do not increase it by more than 5% each time. The super-slow method demands and encourages discipline but the results can often be astonishing, probably because it is better at isolating the muscles being worked.

With the super-slow method the positive phase is 10 instead of 4 seconds

The super-slow method forces you to do the exercise correctly

Advantages of super-slow method:

- corrects poor training habits

- uses full range of motion

- avoids exertion peaks and so protects joints, tendons and ligaments

Use the super-slow method in one of two ways:

1 Use it for several weeks for all exercises. Many who try this method stick with it.

2 Use it solely on those machines where progress has stagnated, that is, you have been unable to increase the weight for some time. In this case train with 20% lower weight for three consecutive sessions. After that return to your normal method and see whether you are now able to increase the weight.

Training records

It is not enough to keep details of your programme "in your head"; they must be recorded on a suitable form. For each session enter the date, which exercises you do and the level of resistance/training weight. The number of repetitions or time under load is useful for clinical purposes but not necessary for preventive training. Reference is also made to this record when you discuss your training with your instructor. Without it trainers would have to rely on assumptions and would be unable to provide expert tuition.

The training card contains a record of all your exercises and the weight used for each exercise

Overtraining

Too much training
makes you weaker

If you do not allow your body time to recover after training strength is reduced rather than increased. The results of too much training are the same as too little: you lose strength.

Signs of overtraining are:

- decline in performance

- loss of weight

- feeling of "exhaustion" when you wake in the morning

- digestive problems

- aversion to foods with protein, e.g., meat and dairy products

- anxiety

- reluctance to train

- susceptibility to colds (immune system!)

If this happens you must stop training immediately for at least 10 days. If your performance then improves significantly this is clear evidence of overtraining.

Therapy

Strength training as a therapy is most successful on patients with chronic back problems, early signs of osteoporosis and general muscular imbalances.

Chronic low back pain

According to leading international orthopaedic specialists, some 80% of all back problems are caused by weak back muscles or to be more precise weak lumbar extensors. The University of Florida was responsible for the pioneering research into the muscular causes of back problems. It was the first to conduct comprehensive research into the theory that weak back muscles could be a cause of chronic low back pain. This research only became possible after the invention of a lumbar extension machine by Arthur Jones. Strength tests conducted on the lower back muscles of several thousand individuals produced some surprising results. The majority—who included highly trained athletes—had weak lumbar extensors. In fact the level of weakness was amazing. However, when these muscles were trained strength levels increased several times over. In fact the level of increase is a clear indication of the level of their previous weakness: the less a muscle is trained the more it can be trained and the greater its potential increase.

After extensive testing, researchers at the University of Florida developed a therapy that achieved spectacular results on patients with chronic back problems.

Patients were given a weekly session of 20 minutes and after 12–18 sessions their pain had disappeared. In order to remain free from pain they only required one session of 5 minutes every 4 weeks. In Europe this procedure is known as Medical Strengthening Therapy (MST) and there are now more than 100 medical practices and clinics in Europe using this

Weak back muscles result in chronic back pain

The less a muscle has been exercised the greater its potential to increase strength and the quicker this happens

Therapy

Transparency of the procedure is vital to win the active co-operation of the patient which in turn is essential for the therapy to succeed

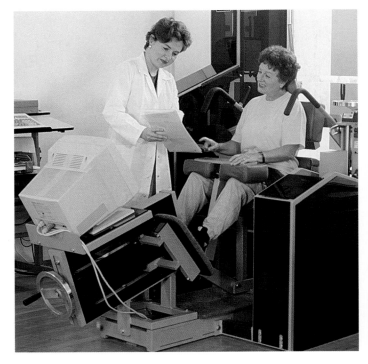

The rotary torso machine is also used to treat back pain.

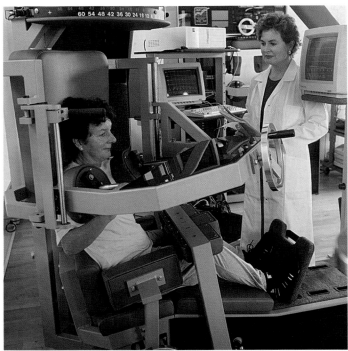

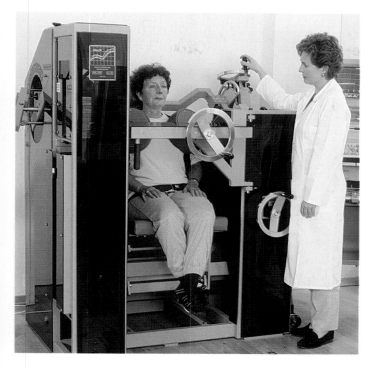

The cervical extension machine treats problems with the cervical spine.

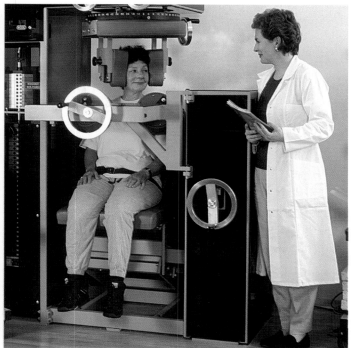

The rotary neck machine is used to strengthen muscles of the head.

Medical strengthening
therapy lasts 12
weeks

technique. Bearing in mind that 50% of those between 30 and 50 suffer from back problems it might be reasonable to assume that the therapy would have caught on very quickly. However, it has not. The strength of the therapy—its effectiveness—is also its weakness, at least as far as speed at which it has caught on. Why?

Back patients are normally long-term patients. They visit their doctor twice a year—normally in the spring and autumn. This provides the medical profession with repeat business and a budgetable and therefore popular source of income. Patients spend money on injections, mud packs, medicinal baths, massage and other measures, all providing further revenue for the medical profession. Although these measures provide patients with temporary relief they are ineffective in the long term.

The therapy is
amazingly successful
on patients with
chronic back
problems

However, MST allows patients to escape from this vicious circle. They disappear from the "back market" and do not reappear.

Osteoporosis

The benefits of strength training are not restricted to muscles. It also rebuilds bones. In conjunction with drugs and dietary changes it is an antidote to a disease suffered by one in three women after the menopause: osteoporosis.

Osteoporosis is loss of bone density. It increases the likelihood of bone fractures. In the USA more women die from the effects of fracturing the neck of the femur than breast and cervical cancer combined. In our latitudes some 12% of the population have X-ray evidence of loss of bone density. With about 25% of women over 60 years old osteoporosis is so far advanced that the spine is deformed.

One in three post-
menopausal women
suffer from
osteoporosis

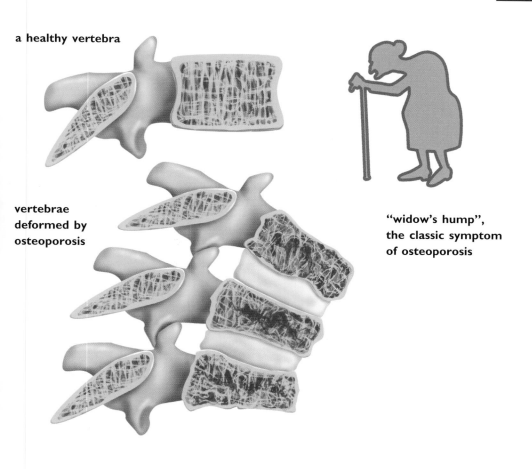

a healthy vertebra

vertebrae deformed by osteoporosis

"widow's hump", the classic symptom of osteoporosis

Although on average fewer men suffer from osteoporosis the number is increasing. Apart from hormonal and dietary factors the lack of muscular strength can play an important role in its development.

Strength training helps to ward off osteoporosis because it develops bones as well as muscles and tendons. Osteoporosis provides the clearest evidence that what we lack most is not movement but strength.

Studies have shown that stamina training is unable to halt osteoporosis, that is, only strength training can reverse the decay.

Strength training is the only effective non-medicinal remedy for osteoporosis

Muscular imbalance

Our entire muscular system is one of interdependence. A change in the strength of one muscle has a knock-on effect on other muscles. Each of us has our own ideal in terms of muscular balance, the right strength relationship between muscles. The degree to which each of us deviates from that ideal varies but the cause is always the same: those muscles subject to loads above the stimulus threshold (trained muscles) as a result of work or leisure activities take the load off other muscles that are much weaker. As a result the latter get weaker and weaker. It is a vicious circle. The resultant imbalance is a very gradual process and at first we do not notice it. It also results in a change in posture. Poor posture is not a bad habit. It is caused by some muscles being stronger than others.

Muscular imbalances are caused by the work you do or the sports you play

Antagonist imbalance

The mechanics of the musculoskeletal system can be likened to the steering on an aircraft. It consists of tension and countertension. An aircraft has an elevator and a rudder (wings and tail) to move up and sideways and we have bones. Aircraft have cables. We have tendons. Despite its simplicity the human system is prone to problems. Muscles, even at rest have a certain level of tension (tone). If the tone in the agonist differs from that in the antagonist the result is a muscle imbalance, that is, different strength levels. Sooner or later this will cause problems.

A muscular imbalance causes problems

Strength training restores that balance by exercising both agonist and antagonist. It would make little sense to stretch only the "shortened" muscle until it was the same strength as its opposite number as that would be a levelling down. What we need to do is to strengthen agonist and antagonist until both reach their strength limit. The weaker muscle soon catches up—the stronger muscle has a much lower growth potential anyway. The closer the two are to their genetic limit the more in balance their strength ratio.

Inter-muscular imbalance

Another type of muscular imbalance is the one found in a chain of muscles. Normally any given movement requires a cooperative effort by several muscles in a so-called chain. If the work required for a specific movement involves several muscles the relationship between the strengths of these muscles must be right. If not the result is an inter-muscular imbalance. To eliminate this imbalance we need to isolate the weaker muscle and then strengthen it. If the muscle is not isolated the stronger muscle will come to the "aid" of the weaker one. Once the muscle has reached its ideal strength the muscles are in balance. Experience has shown that once restored the balance can usually be maintained without further training. This is because the new strength ratio changes our posture and the way we move and so the work is distributed more evenly between the muscles.

If muscles fail to work in harmony this is known as an inter-muscular imbalance

Those with chronic low back pain are normally suffering from an inter-muscular imbalance. Most of the work to straighten the back is done by two muscle groups: the gluteus maximus and the back extensors. The latter also include the so-called autochthonous back muscles of the spine. In most cases our back extensors are weaker than our gluteus maximus. Unfortunately we unconsciously change our posture and the way we move allowing the gluteus muscle to take on more and more of the work of the back extensors. As a result the latter lack stimulus and become weaker and weaker, a vicious circle. It can only be broken if back extensors are isolated and strengthened: we need to exclude the gluteals.

We tend to transfer load from the weaker to the stronger muscle

Intra-muscular imbalance

However, the most common form of imbalance is one within a muscle, that is an intra-muscular imbalance. Even amongst professionals it is still largely unknown because the tools required to diagnose it are relatively new. Unlike the other two types this imbalance is in the muscle itself rather than in the relationship between individual muscles. An intra-muscular imbalance is caused by the normal stresses and strains put on muscles during our work and play. These activities only work (train) a fraction of our full range of motion.

More recently, standard data on the strength required by a muscle throughout the various angles of a movement have become available, at least for the lumbar and cervical regions.

Even amongst specialist intra-muscular balance remains almost unknown

Growing field of applications

Reports from the United States indicate that medical strengthening therapy on neck muscles has been successful in the treatment of certain jaw problems. Ongoing research is clearly opening up new areas where strength training can be effective. We should not be surprised at this: as strength grows so do we, as strength withers so do we. Instead of strength we have pain. As a result we avoid further exertions and so become even weaker.

For example if a shoulder is not immobilized after an injury, recovery time is 18 days. If immobilized for 7 days recovery time is 52 days, if immobilized for 14 days recovery time is 121 days and if immobilized for 21 days recovery time is 300 days (*Journal of Bone and Joint Surgery*, 1953; 35B: 521–539).

The areas where strength training can be effective continue to increase

Case study

Actual and ideal strength curves at start of therapy: the patient is 49 years old, a medical doctor, water-skier and she suffered chronic back pain radiating down to her legs for years. She completed 18 sessions on the MedX lumbar extension machine and is now free from pain. An interesting feature of this example is the S-shaped

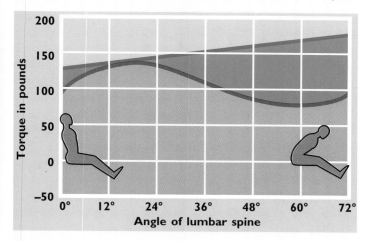

strength curve of the first test. It is indicative of the patient's sport. Water-skiing puts a load on lower back muscles, that is, muscles are trained in the position where the graph shows the patient is strongest. The straight line above is the ideal strength curve.

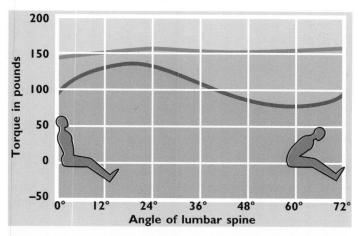

Strength curves at start of therapy (lower) and at the end (upper). Overall strength has improved considerably, the intra-muscular imbalance is largely eliminated and the pain has disappeared.

Supplementary action

"What else can I do?"—a perennial question from many seeking to accelerate progress. What never ceases to amaze me is the willingness of some, at least verbally, to change their lifestyle in any number of ways: change their diet or sleeping habits, learn and play a range of sports or other new activity as a complement to strength training. Behind this sometimes quite sudden unrest is a desire to be someone quite different, an ideal version as it were of what they are in reality. What is more they want to achieve it quickly.

You cannot accelerate biological processes. However, you can retard them

However that is not how things work. Biological processes take time. You have lived with your genetic makeup up to now and you will have to live with it in the future. You are what you are. However, you can, as we have seen, influence a fundamental element of quality of life: strength. To exert that influence you need to train and display a certain degree of persistence. Nothing else is required. Of course you need a so-called balanced diet, enough sleep and a psychosocial environment where you feel at ease. However, apart from incorporating two training sessions into your weekly timetable no other changes are required.

But it is worth explaining a few points in a little more detail—not as a way of accelerating progress but to ensure that progress is not impeded by some other deficit.

Diet

The trained body holds more water than an untrained one

There is a considerable body of literature available on the subject of diet and an understanding of our requirements in terms of protein, fat, carbohydrate, vitamins, minerals and trace elements is almost common knowledge. Strength training does not require a special diet, either in terms of quantity or quality.

In contrast water is particularly important for strength training. Muscles are 70–80% water. The more a muscle is exercised the greater its water content. During training your peripherals, particularly muscles need more water. Consequently it is important to drink more during and after training even if you are not thirsty. Our perception of thirst is not always a reliable indicator of what we need. Wherever possible drink cold water, particularly if you want to lose weight. Cold water takes calories from the body. The actual volume of water required depends of course on air temperature but based on average temperatures in much of Europe the daily adult requirement is some 30 ml/kg. Too much water does no harm but too little quickly causes serious damage.

Cold water takes calories from the body

With red wine the opposite is true. Nevertheless the daily recommendation is still one (1!) glass. In fact recent research has shown that this can reduce the danger of circulatory problems.

If you want to lose weight, simply reduce the carbohydrate content of what you eat and increase the protein. It is important to continue training during a diet as otherwise you lose muscle instead of fat.

To lose weight restrict your carbohydrate intake

UV rays

UV rays seem to encourage the development of strength. In a double-blind trial the reduced trainability of muscles in winter was increased to summer levels when test subjects were exposed to regular UV light therapy. However, this only happened if the rays were erythemogenic, that is, produced a slight reddening of the skin but not sunburn. The machines used in commercial suntan studios are not suitable for this purpose because they produce a tan. They do not redden the skin.

Sunlight, correctly dispensed, can aid training

Clothing

Clothing is designed to protect us from the cold and undue exposure to UV sunlight. Training clothes must not restrict movement in any way. Tight clothing reduces the circulation of air on the surface of the skin.

Sports shoes with a thick sole restrict ankle movements. They give stability to a joint whereas it is muscles that should be providing this stability. If worn regularly these shoes weaken the muscles that move the ankle. Similarly, normal gym shoes are unsuitable as they impede heat dispersal. The ideal is a thin gym shoe, apparatus footwear or sandals such as "Clarks" or "Birkenstock". They allow the joint to move without restriction and the foot can give off heat freely.

Clothing should be as light as possible. Wear thin materials, if possible cotton or silk. Avoid thick track-suits or skin-tight bodies. The aim is to get rid of heat not trap it. Elasticated garments prevent air circulating between the surface of the body and your clothes. They also cling making them feel unpleasant. To prevent trousers slipping just use a tie-cord or similar in the waistband. Trousers should rest on the hips. They should not constrict the stomach as this can impede breathing. Colours have a psychological effect. Bright colours make you feel more cheerful and dark ones more sombre. Physical exertion alters the way the body distributes heat. Some parts of the body may receive too little heat compared with others. There are two critical areas that must be covered at all times: shoulders and kidneys. Both are sensitive to draughts and cold. Cold makes shoulders more susceptible to rheumatic ailments and kidneys more prone to infection. Clothing for the upper body should be long at the back, loose at the neck and cover arms as far as the elbows.

Exercise alters the
normal pattern of
heat distribution

Body-awareness

This means training methods such as those developed by Feldenkrais and Alexander, which increase your understanding of the body and so increase self-awareness. If you find it difficult to isolate certain muscles during training it may help to take a course in one of these techniques. All major towns have therapists offering such courses.

Improved body-awareness aids training

Instructing strength training as a profession

Most instructors working in health and fitness clubs have a sports background, both in terms of theory and practice. However sports training and strength training have quite different objectives. Sport is the use and consumption of strength for the purpose of winning. Health is secondary and amongst the sporting elite it is of no importance at all. They regard strength training merely as a preparation for their particular sport.

In contrast health-oriented strength training is not designed to enhance performance but to maximize our efficiency in dealing with the laws of physics. This difference must be reflected in the education and training given to instructors. If the emphasis is on performance, as is typical with most courses, this will inevitably reduce the quality of the strength-training exercises and so reduce their effect.

In addition health-oriented strength training is not restricted to the relatively small sporting community. It is targeted at a very much larger group, "normal" people with other jobs and few sporting ambitions. It is targeted at those whose main interest is not physical exercise but a desire to maintain a healthy body.

However, there are strength trainers who are also qualified doctors, physiotherapists or come from another medical profession and this can often be a problem. Although their training, including the training given to doctors, contains little on strength development, some of them harbour a strange prejudice. It manifests itself in statements such as "I know about that already". A more appropriate comment would be "I ought to know about that". To accept strength training as a therapy requires a fundamental change in medicine. Professional therapists are all too willing to regard strength training as an addition to their existing procedures. However, in reality strength training renders some of their procedures obsolete. Unfortunately they are reluctant to give them up for employ-

An emphasis on performance reduces the effect of strength training

Strength training is not included in the training given to the medical profession

ment reasons. In addition most therapists only have contact with those who are unwell and so tend to apply the principle of rest and inactivity even when it is not appropriate, for instance, in the case of chronic back pain. What one person perceives as muscular pain another will perceive as minor muscle stiffness combined with a pleasant feeling of "having done something". This means that strength training therapists must have personal experience of strength training. Only then can they distinguish between "good" and "bad" pain. In other words all therapists must also train.

All trainers, irrespective of educational background and whether they are involved in the preventive or therapy side of strength training, must complete further training. Moreover this training must be both comprehensive and standard.

Strength trainers working on the therapy side must do strength training themselves

Encouraging independence not dependence

A trainer once announced proudly that "his" customers liked to come to him. They were even reluctant to train if he was not there. To his amazement I said he was doing something fundamentally wrong.

In fact many trainers believe they must motivate customers (or pupils) by showering them with praise or other rewards. Certainly a friendly and understanding attitude is preferable to a sullen one. However, with this method of extrinsic motivation you are constantly having to invent new and more powerful incentives as the value of each incentive quickly diminishes. This method cultivates a dependence on the trainer that ultimately puts an undue load on the trainer. This is the main reason why many instructors complain of "burn-out". A so-called personal trainer

Some trainers foster an attitude of dependence amongst customers

once complained that he constantly had to think up new "tricks" for customers in order to maintain their motivation. His efforts to encourage self-reliance failed because customers valued the concept of "total care". After all it was what they were paying for.

When training animals, extrinsic motivation is the only option available. An animal is not capable of the independent thought process required for intrinsic motivation. Even the process of instilling fear is a part of extrinsic motivation.

A "master" instructor is someone who can ignite a passion in the minds of students that is both sustained and self-sustaining. In short: a successful instructor makes himself superfluous because he can activate a permanent state of intrinsic motivation in the minds of students.

Good instructors generate intrinsic motivation in their clients

Job satisfaction as an instructor

The training given to strength instructors must include intrinsic motivation, the origin of the concept and its development. Strength training, unlike skiing, tennis and other leisure activities with a physical emphasis, does not bring immediate pleasure. Strength training can only survive as a concept if the need for it is understood. The role of a responsible instructor is to ensure that this understanding becomes firmly embedded in the minds of customers, that is, it becomes part of their moral code.

Instead of constantly offering something new it is better to return repeatedly to basics

Rather than constantly offering something new it means returning time and time to basics, that is, repetition. This is not only less strenuous for the instructor but also more satisfying. It allows students to free themselves from the instructor. The seed, once sown, starts to grow. The instructor has instilled in them something that will sustain them throughout their life. Fallacies are passed down from generation to gener-

Fallacies and prejudices

ation whereas prejudices are created by each new generation. We rarely question statements once they have been made. The following list contains a few of the fallacies and prejudices prevalent in the area of strength training and in body culture in general.

'Strength training is sport'

1 Sport is the use and consumption of strength in a game or competition. Strength training is the development and maintenance of the musculoskeletal system so that it continues to work properly.

2 'Strength training is more dangerous than other activities'

Productive strength training is strenuous and subjects the body to load peaks. Any existing health problems may, therefore, become acute. If you have any doubts about your health consult a doctor before taking it up. This recommendation is not at variance with the fact that, provided you are in good health, strength training done properly is almost risk-free. The same cannot be said for most sports. Even everyday activities such as moving quickly from a standing to a crouching position subjects the body to load peaks and exposes it to risks not encountered with strength training done correctly. If problems arise with strength training this is the result of either latent health problems, which show up prematurely when the body is put under load or "accelerated" or even "explosive" movements, similar to those which, stupidly, are still recommended as preparation for sport.

If you are healthy strength training is not dangerous

3 'Sweating cleans and purifies'

Sweating has only one purpose: it cools the surface of the body to prevent overheating. It does not protect you from colds and does not "clean out" the pores. Similarly it does not help elimi-

It is a fallacy that sweating is healthy

nate toxins or waste products (there are none). If you sweat profusely your muscles are particularly vulnerable because they are more than 70% water and you can lose strength. To avoid overheating during training avoid excessively warm clothing. The ideal room temperature for strength training is less than 20 degrees Celsius.

4 **'Each type of sports needs its own strength training'**

This is only true in as much as you select those exercises that work most in a particular sport. However, it is wrong to imitate a movement, in a particular sport, but to do it under an increased load, for example, doing the high jump wearing a waistcoat filled with weights, a sprint start against an elastic resistance, running with "heavy-hand" dumb-bells, doing the shot-putt with an overweight shot, etc. This type of exercise creates new memory patterns, which differ, even if only slightly, from the original movement. You then run the risk that you will make a mistake in actual competition. When practising the movements required for a particular sport you should mimic the conditions that prevail in actual competition. In other words the best practice for a footballer is to play football and for skier it is to ski, etc.

In the last 15 years I have trained hundreds of competitive athletes, some of them top-class including at least 20 Olympic medallists and world champions in sports as diverse as shooting, bobsleigh, downhill skiing, speed skating, tennis, judo, karate, cycling, riding, and motor cycling. However, the differences in training programmes have only been minor. The training principles have always been identical: from big to small muscles, slow movements and a low training volume.

It is foolish to do movements for a specific sport against a resistance

5 'If I do strength training movements fast it will make me faster'

Fast movements are dangerous and unproductive in strength training. Dangerous because load peaks occur in the deceleration phase and this can easily result in tendon fractures. Unproductive because the duration of load peaks is too short to create a stimulus and the rest of the movement, that is, the acceleration of the weight (momentum), puts no load on the muscle.

Trainers who recommend that those under their supervision jump off a table or bench with a weight over and above their body weight, should be prosecuted.

In strength training rapid movements are both dangerous and unproductive

6 'The last repetition is dangerous'

No, the first is dangerous if there is not a conscious effort to do it slowly. When you start your muscles are still fresh and strong and can produce a high level of tension immediately. When you do the final repetitions the muscles are too weak to do any damage. However, the final repetitions or seconds are what counts. This is when you exceed the so-called stimulus threshold.

The stimulus occurs in the final seconds of an exercise

7 'First muscle mass then definition'

Muscle mass creates definition. The greater the muscle mass the more contoured the body looks. Muscle mass is often compared to a block of marble shaped (defined) by the sculptor. This is an incorrect analogy. Fat cannot be chiselled out, at best it can be removed if you go hungry. In addition you cannot target where you lose weight. The claim that you can lose weight exactly where you want to is nonsense. Where you put on or lose weight depends upon genetic makeup.

Aching muscles are a harmless temporary phenomenon.

8 **'Aching muscles are caused by lactic acid'**

Aching muscles are a transient inflammatory phenomenon caused by minute tears in muscle fibre and although harmless can be annoying. These minute tears occur during the extension of a muscle under a high load (going down hill) not during contraction. Stretching and applying heat or ointment cannot prevent or alleviate aching muscles.

More strength allows you to move more quickly

9 **'Strong muscles slow you down'**

Speed of movement depends primarily on strength and coordination, your level of skill. If muscles are strong movements can be faster provided you also have good coordination. If you lack coordination you cannot use your strength. However, it does not slow you down.

10 **'Strong muscles make you less flexible'**

Even extremely large muscles do not impede flexibility, quite the reverse. The range of motion under load is greater if you have strong muscles. In other words strength training done correctly increases flexibility.

Our diet contains more than enough protein

11 **'Protein concentrates are essential for strength training'**

Muscle growth only needs slightly more protein than normal. In most of the developed world average protein intake is far higher than what we actually need. In other words there is no risk of protein deficiency. Much more important is the need for more water. Muscles are 70% water and metabolic processes—including muscle build-up—require an abundant supply of water.

12

'Women should train differently from men'

In qualitative (if not quantitative) terms female muscles are intrinsically the same as male muscles. Insofar as they are subject to the same physiological laws. There is no reason, therefore, why women should train differently.

13

'Stomach exercises combat a spare tyre'

The only way to lose weight is to use more calories than you consume. Where you lose weight depends on your genetic makeup and any fat that happens to be near the muscle being exercised is largely unaffected. Exercises for the stomach muscles produce the same weight loss as exercises for the gluteals.

Exercises have no effect on localized fat deposits

14

'Provided you have the determination you can succeed in any sport'

You cannot "make" an athlete but you can make an athlete better. It is your genetic make-up that decides whether you are athletic.

You may be quite determined to become a world-class basketball player. However, if you have the misfortune to be only 165 cm tall no amount of determination will help and you will be ignored on the field of play. Even in the narrower field of power sport there are enormous differences. For example the physical proportions required for weightlifters are quite different from those required for bodybuilders.

Top sporting performances have more to do with genetic make-up and less with training

Ideal weightlifter	Ideal bodybuilder
Short legs	Long legs
Short arms	Long arms
Long torso	Short torso
Narrow shoulders	Broad shoulders
Broad hips	Narrow hips

If each were to increase muscle mass by 10 kg this would make a better weightlifter and a better bodybuilder. However, no training in the world will turn a bodybuilder into an ideal weightlifter and vice-versa.

15 'Trained muscles are unnatural'
A muscle does not know why it reacts. Muscle reaction is the same irrespective of whether the tension that produces a stimulus comes from training or heavy physical labour.

16 'If you stop training muscles become "flabby"'
If the muscle is not subject to normal tension it loses mass as surely as a muscle builds up mass when tension is increased, the film just rewinds. However, when you then restart training the build-up process is accelerated.

17 'Training to music aids progress'
Music improves coordination (for example dance). The sole purpose of coordination is to prevent undue strain during a specific movement. However, with strength training the aim is not to complete a set of precise movements. Its aim is to subject muscles to tension stimuli. Although the exercise needs a certain rhythm it may not be the same rhythm as that of the music. Music tempts you to do elegant exercises. However, an exercise is only elegant if it requires no effort.

18 'Strength training is not suitable for children'
Children may and should do strength training. Strength training helps dampen the dangerous spurts in growth that can occur during adolescence. The Orthopaedic Clinic at the University of California uses strength training to treat children with scoliosis

(spinal deviations). However, children may have a problem because of their height. To use most machines you need to be at least 1.5 metres tall. If strength training were part of physical education at school it would be worth making smaller machines.

Strength training can correct spinal deviations in children

19 'More strength yes, more muscle no!'

Increases in strength are linear. Increases in mass are spasmodic and so before each spurt there is actually an increase in strength without a corresponding increase in muscle mass. However, this has nothing to do with training methods. It is merely what happens when strength/mass is increased significantly. In fact a major long-term increase in muscle strength without an associated increase in mass would be a biological perpetuum mobile.

Increase in strength without increases in mass would be a biological perpetuum mobile

The process works this way because our body has an efficient energy management system. Before the body allows an increase in mass, something that requires considerable energy, it rationalizes what is going on in the muscle. This is known as intra-muscular coordination. However, if the load is then increased further it has to increase mass in order to respond to the demand.

20 'Before starting strength training you must do some sport'

The opposite is true: It is dangerous to play a sport without the necessary muscular infrastructure; first strengthen muscles and with them bones and tendons as well. Strength training is build-up. Sport is consumption.

21 'There are various types of strength'

The ability of a muscle to contract creates tension. This tension is used as a measurement of strength. In this respect it does not matter whether the tension is more, less or the same as the resistance that it overcomes, gives in to or simply withstands. If strength increases, that is, there is an increase in the ability of the muscle to contract, the muscle is faster (resistance as a function of speed) and has more stamina (anaerobic). It acquires the properties that can be acquired with training. Of course there are many other factors that influence muscle performance, for example, leverage ratio (determined by tendon attachments), distribution of "fast" and "slow" fibres, etc. However, these factors are immutable because they are determined by our genetic makeup.

Irrespective of the strength we require the training remains the same. It makes no difference to the muscle how we use our acquired strength. If a stimulus occurs a muscle develops. If a stimulus does not occur, a muscle does not develop. There is no more to say!

Although strength may manifest itself in many forms the training is the same

22 'Muscle shape and firm muscles'

Muscles can adapt: if demand on them is increased they increase in size (hypertrophy), if demand is reduced they reduce in size (atrophy). That is it. You cannot lengthen or shorten muscles and you cannot thicken part of them. A muscle is firm because it has increased its overall size following an increase in osmotic pressure resulting from an intake of water.

23 'Training with free weights aids coordination'

Coordination skills are specific; they are tailored to individual activities. They are not transferable. In other words the sense of balance acquired by doing squats with barbells is of no help when skiing or cycling. The balance required on the slopes or on the bike can only be acquired by skiing or cycling.

Training with barbells develops a form of coordination that can only be used for barbell training

24 'We suffer from a lack of movement'

It is not movement we lack but strength. Without strength muscles, tendons and bones disappear and in the end so do we. When we talk about the need for more movement we should add the words "against what?" The term "lack of movement " implies that we need to exercise as much as possible. This explains the vague and somewhat distracted nature of many fitness activities. Frenzy is equated with activity.

Exercise is only good if done against a resistance

25 'Stretching prevents injury'

There is currently no conclusive evidence that stretching can prevent injuries or aching muscles. Similarly there is no proof that stretching every 2 hours prevents stiff muscles after exercise. Tests have also shown that those who stretch before exercising muscles to the point of local fatigue experienced the same degree of muscle ache as those who had not stretched. In contrast stretching can result in hypermobility of joints, a form of permanent damage to the musculoskeletal system. Machine-based training done correctly automatically provides the level of movement prescribed by nature for a particular muscle.

Stretching cannot prevent injuries

26 'Strength training is only for younger people'

Older people benefit more from strength training than younger people. This is because it slows down the degenerative processes that accelerate with age allowing regenerative processes to

Strength training helps older people retard the degenerative processes that affect the body

flourish, for example the ability of strength training to promote the restructuring of bone tissue.

27 **'Lower training intensity aids weight loss'**
Until recently this was thought to be true. However, recent research tends to indicate the opposite. Fat reserves are attacked more quickly if training is short but highly intensive.

Bibliography

Amirfallah N., Baum E.: Die Auswirkungen dynamischen Krafttrainings auf Kardiozirkulatorische Parameter, Weimar 1995

Berger R.: Effect of varied weight training programs on strength. *Res. Q* 1962; **33**:168–81.

Brooks G.A., Fahey T.D.: Exercise Physiology: Human Bioenergetics and its Applications, New York: Macmillan 1984

Brück K., Olschewsky H.: Human Acclimation, Body Temperature and Endurance Performance, Odense 1988

Brück K.: Warmlaufen oder Kaltstart? Sportliche Höchstleistungen durch Kälte, Gießen 1987

Carpenter D.: Effect of 12 and 20 weeks of resistance training on lumbar extension torque production, Gainesville 1991

Darden E.: The Nautilus Diet: ten weeks to a Brand New Body, Boston: Little Brown & Company 1987

Darden E.: The Nautilus Book, Chicago: Contemporary Books, 1990

Deutsche Gesellschaft für Ernährung: Empfehlungen für die Nährstoffzufuhr, Frankfurt 1995

Dubs R.: Sportmedizin für Jedermann, Zürich 1954

Feldenkrais M.: Der aufrechte Gang. Tel-Aviv 1967

Fiatarone M.: High-Intensity Strength Training in Nonagenarians, Boston 1990

Gotshalk L.A., Loebel C.C., Nindl B.C. et al.: Hormonal responses of multiset versus single-set heavy-resistance exercise protocols, *Can J Appl. Physiol* 1997; **22**: 244–55.

Graves J.E. et al.: Single versus multiple set dynamic and isometric lumbar extension strength training. Proceedings, Book III, World Confederation for Physical Therapy, 11th International Congress, London: United Kingdom, 1991, pp. 1340–1342.

Hackenschmidt G.: Der Weg zur Kraft, Leipzig ca. 1910

Häkkinen K.: Neuromuscular and hormonal adaptions during strength and power training: a review. *J Sports Med Phys Fitness* 1989; **29**: 9–26

Herz M.: Lehrbuch der Heilgymnastik, Berlin 1903

Hettinger Th.: Isometrisches Muskeltraining, Stuttgart 1964

Hoster M.: (Hrsg.) Dehnen und Mobilisieren, Waldenburg 1993

Jahn L.: Die Deutsche Turnkunst, Berlin 1960

Jones A.: The lumbar spine, the cervical spine and the knee, Ocala 1993

Jones A.: Bulletin No. 1, DeLand 1970

Jones A.: Bulletin No. 2, DeLand 1971

Josenhans W.T.: An evaluation of some methods of improving muscle strength. *Rev Canad Biol* 1962; **21**.

Kieser W.: Vom Krafttraining zur Krafttherapie, Zürich 1990

Kieser W.: Hanteltraining zu Hause, Niedernhausen 1993

Kieser W.: Kiesers Krafttraining an Maschinen, Niedernhausen 1993

Kieser W.: Krafttraining, Niedernhausen 1996

Kieser W.: Die Seele der Muskeln, Zürich 1997

Kieser W.: Wieviele Sätze beim Krafttraining? Frankfurt 1998

Kraemer W.J.: Endokrine Reaktionen und

Bibliography

Adaptionen unter einem Krafttraining. Kraft und Schnellkraft im Sport. Köln 1994

Kreck H.C.: Die Medico-Mechanische Therapie Gustav Zanders in Deutschland, Frankfurt a. M. 1987

Kuznezow W.W.: Kraftvorbereitung. Theoretische Grundlagen der Muskelkraftentwicklung, Moskau 1970

Lukas G.: Die Körperkultur in frühen Epochen, Berlin 1969

Mooney V.: On the Dose of Therapeutic Exercise, San Diego 1994

Morehouse L.E.: Physiological Basis of Strength Development, New York 1960

Müller E.A., Rohmert W.: Die Geschwindigkeit der Muskelkraftzunahme bei isometrischem *Training. Int. Z. angew. Physiol.* 19, 1963

Müller K.-J.: Statische und dynamische Muskelkraft. Beiträge zur Sportwissenschaft. Bd. 7. Frankfurt/Main 1987

Nelson B.W.: The Clinical Effects of Intensive Specific Exercise on Chronic Low Back Pain, Columbia 1995

Peterson J.A.: The Effect of High Intensity Weight Training on Cardiovascular Function, Westpoint 1976

Pollock M.L., Graves J. E., Bamman M.M. et al.: Frequency and volume of resistance training: effect of cervical extension strength. *Arch. Phys. Med. Rehabil.* 1993; **74:**1080–86.

Pollock M., Graves J.: New Approach to Low Back Evaluation and Training, Gainesville 1989

Pollock M.: Effects of Isolated Lumbar Extension Resistance Training on Bone Mineral Density, Indianapolis 1991

Riemkasten F.: Die Alexander-Methode, Heidelberg 1967

Rohen J. W.: Funktionelle Anatomie des Menschen, Stuttgart 1993

Rouet M.: Toute la Culture Physique, Paris 1965

Silvester L.: The effect of variable resistance and free weight training programms on strength and vertical jump. *Nat. Strength Condit. J.* 1982; **3:**30-33.

Starkey D.B., Pollock M.L., Ishida Y. et al.: Effect of resistance training volume on strength and muscle thickness. *Med Sci Sport Exerc* 1996; **28**: 1311–20.

Stevens Ch.: Alexander Technik, Ein Weg zum besseren Umgang mit sich selbst, Basel 1989

Stoll T., Brühlmann P., Michel B. A.: Assessment of Muscle Strength in Poly-Dermatomyositis (PM/DM): Validation of a New, Simple, Quantitative Method, Zürich 1993

Stowers T. et al.: The short-term effect of three different strength-power training methods. *Nat. Strength Condit. J.* 1983; **5:**24–27.

Webster D.: Barbells + Beefcake, Portsmouth 1979

Westcott W. L.: Strength Fitness. Physiological Principles and Training Techniques, Dubuque 1995

Westcott W. L.: Four key factors in building a strength program. *Scholastic Coach* 1986; **55:**104–5.

Westcott W. L. et al.: Strength-training research: sets & repetitions. *Scholastic Coach* 1989; **58:**98–100.

Index

Index

Index

Index